SEX, PORN AND MASTURBATION ADDICTION MASTERY: A COMPREHENSIVE PRACTICAL GUIDE TO RE-FOCUSING YOUR SEXUAL ENERGY

Identifying, Solving and Recovering from Sexual and Love Addictions

DAVID WHITEHEAD

Silk Publishing

INTRODUCTION

Sex addiction is a subject that should be discussed

— CAREY MULLIGAN, AUTHOR: *GIRLS &
BOYS*

Every addict comes to a point in his or her life when the consequences are so severe, or the pain is so excruciating that the addict admits his or her sexual behavior has taken control of his or her life. Some are newsworthy, such as when a congressman, minister, or professional figure is chastised for unacceptable sexual behavior. Millions of people read the steamy news accounts and, despite their lust, pass harsh judgment on people who are sexual with children, visit prostitutes, commit homosexual acts in public restrooms, or even have affairs. A smaller but far larger audience read each line, fearful that the same public exposure would happen to them and judging themselves with the same unforgiving standards as the public.

Some are dramatic moments, like:

- When the cop car pulls into your driveway, and you know why they've come...
- When you end yet another relationship that you never wanted to be in...
- When your spouse declares the end of your marriage due to the most recent discovery...
- When your daughter's friend sees your picture in the police station mug shots, and no one in your family knows...
- When you have to leave your job because of a sexual entanglement with a person you never really liked anyway . . .
- When your teenage son finds your pornography . . .
- When the school counselor phones to say, your daughter won't come home because she doesn't want to be sexual after eight years, and you are being referred to child protection...
- When you're in a car accident while exposing yourself.

Some are secret moments known only to yourself, like:

- When you're forced to say yet another lie that you almost believe yourself...
- When the money you have spent on the last prostitute equals the amount for the new shoes your child needs . . .
- When you run into someone on the street, and the person is someone you have had a sexual encounter with in a restroom.

- When you make business travel decisions not based on the company interests, but rather the affair that you are having . . .

- When you tell someone "I love you," knowing full well, there are two others who also think they are the only ones you love . . .

- When you sit in a room full of people, three of whom you have made love with recently. Part of you fears what they would do if they knew, and part of you gloats over your accomplishment . . .

- When you say "I love you" because you know you will go to bed with someone. Yet you don't love him, nor do you want to go to bed with him . . .

- When you cringe inside because your friends are laughing at a flasher joke, and you are one . . .

- When you are an alcoholic completing treatment, and you realize that your time in the hospital was a period free from chemicals and a time when you were sexually at ease as well, and you never felt better. You know, however, that sobriety will be easy compared to stopping your sexual addiction.

For most people, these moments are followed by resolves "never to do it again." Even as the promises are made, they are rendered hollow by the echoes of the previous vows and resolutions. Many addicts have profoundly wished not to be sexual, thinking that to be the only cure for their compulsive feelings, thinking that by giving up their sexuality, they would be able to work, love, and enjoy themselves like other people. Sexual addiction has been referred to as "the athlete's foot of the mind." It doesn't go away. It always begs to be scratched, as if it would bring relief. However, to scratch is to cause pain and intensify the itch.

The "itch" is created partly by the rationalizations, lies, and beliefs about themselves carried deep within the sexual addicts. For example, the husband visits a prostitute and, on his way home, feels warmly towards his wife and family, tells himself that his time in the sauna really helps him be more sensitive and loving to his family. At one level, he knows the fallacy of his thinking but chooses to ignore it in light of the immediate warm feelings. In contrast with the unfeeling exchanges of massage parlor life, the family does look much better. The cost to the family remains overlooked, however. So it is with the many beliefs, rationalizations, and myths that support addiction:

- I am oversexed.
- No one else is like me.
- I really did care for her/him.
- Just one more time won't hurt.
- I deserve it.
- It isn't so bad since everyone does it.

One of the most common misconceptions that causes an addict to repeat sexual behaviors is that it has no negative effect on other relationships, especially a marriage. In fact, an addict will say, "I do it to stay in the marriage."

This is one of the most popular rationales for a married addict.

In reality, though, the marriage is often characterized by diminishing intimacy, sensitivity, and sexuality. The corollary myth is that the family does not know about the secret sexual life. Yet, at one level, they always do know... even the children.

So if you are reading this book, know that you're at the right place to find solutions to your sexual addiction. The primary aim of this book is to assist people who struggle with compulsive and addictive sexual behaviors by assisting them in recognizing their problem as a chronic emotional condition and understanding that, like alcoholism, compulsive gambling, eating disorders, and opioid abuse, the problem can be placed into remission with proper treatment and guidance.

In a nutshell, this book reassures those suffering from sexual addiction that their sexual needs can be treated without stigma or moral/cultural/religious prejudice. Most of all, it offers sex addicts hope, letting them know that long-term change and healing are possible for anyone willing to invest in the hard work of personal growth and integrity. So, keep calm, and let's begin!

UNDERSTANDING THE BASICS
OF SEXUAL ADDICTION
WHAT IS SEX ADDICTION?

Sexual addiction, also called hyper-sexuality, hypersexual disorder, and sexual compulsivity, is a behavioral addiction focused on sex and sexual fantasy. More specifically, sex addiction is a dysfunctional preoccupation with sexual urges, fantasies, and behaviors, often involving the obsessive pursuit of objectified non-intimate sexuality: pornography, casual/anonymous sex, prostitution, etc. This adult pattern of sexual urges, fantasies, and behaviors must continue for at least six months, despite related negative life consequences and (failed) attempts to either stop or curtail the pleasurable but problem-inducing behaviors. In short, sex addiction is an ongoing, out-of-control pattern of compulsive sexual fantasies and behaviors that causes problems in the addict's life.

The consequences of sexual addiction can be quite varied in nature. For instance, a recent United Kingdom survey of 350 self-identified sex addicts found that sex addicts commonly experience the following problems:

- Shame
- Low self-esteem
- Mental Health Issue
- Loss of a Relationship
- Sexual Dysfunction
- Serious Suicidality
- Sexually Transmitted Disease
- Other (Non-STD) Physical Health Problems
- Debt
- Impaired Parenting
- Loss of Employment
- Press Exposure

Like other addicts, sex addicts typically abuse both fantasy and behavior as ways to "numb out" and escape from stress and emotional (and sometimes physical) discomfort—including the pain of underlying emotional and psychological issues like depression, anxiety, early-life trauma, abandonment fears and the like. In other words, sex addicts don't use compulsive sexual fantasies and behaviors to feel better; they use them to distract themselves from what they are feeling at that moment. As such, sexual addiction is not about having fun; no matter how good the sex itself, it's about controlling (by escaping) what one feels.

In sum, sex addicts are hooked on the dissociative euphoria produced by intense sexual fantasies and directly related patterns of sexual behavior (including their "endless" search for sex). They typically find as much excitement and escape in fantasizing about and searching for their next sexual encounter as in the sex act itself. Thus they can spend hours, sometimes even days, in this elevated emotional state —high on the goal/idea of having sex—before actually engaging in any concrete sexual act. Because of this, sex addicts spend much more time engaged in the fantasy and ritualized pursuit of sex than in the sex act itself.

Patterns of problematic fantasy-driven behavior typically exhibited by sex addicts often include:

- Compulsive use of pornography, with or without masturbation
- Compulsive use of one or more digital "sexnologies," i.e., webcams, sexting, dating/hookup websites and hook-up apps, virtual reality sex games, sexual devices, etc.
- Consistently being "on the hunt" for sexual activity
- Multiple affairs or brief "serial" relationships
- Consistent involvement with strip clubs, adult bookstores, adult movie theaters, sex clubs, and other sex-focused environments
- Ongoing involvement with prostitution or sensual massage (hiring or providing)
- A pattern of anonymous or casual sexual hookups with people met online via apps, websites, or in person
- Repeatedly engaging in unprotected sex
- Repeatedly engaging in sex with potentially dangerous people or in potentially dangerous places

- Seeking sexual experiences without regard to immediate or long-term potential consequences
- In some, repeated patterns of minor sexual offenses such as voyeurism, exhibitionism, frotteurism, etc.

COMMON SIGNS AND SYMPTOMS OF SEXUAL ADDICTION

Regardless of age, race, gender, social history, or psychological underpinnings, the core signs and symptoms of sexual addiction are largely the same. In fact, almost all sex addicts report, in some form or another, the following:

Obsessive Sexual Fantasy and Preoccupation

Sex addicts are obsessed with romance and sex. They fantasize about it, plan for it, pursue it, and engage in it for hours, if not days. The majority of their choices are influenced by sex, including what they wear, the car they drive, which gym they attend, their relationships, and possibly even their career path.

Loss of Control

Sex addicts lose control of their ability to decline sexual fantasies and habits. They make promises to themselves or others to quit or cut back, but they keep failing.

Related Adverse Consequences

Sex addicts eventually face the same basic negative life consequences as alcoholics, drug addicts, compulsive gamblers, compulsive spenders, and all other addicts, such as job loss, academic difficulties, financial difficulties, ruined relationships, declining physical or emotional health, loss of interest in previously enjoyable activities, loss of time, isolation, arrest, and so on.

Tolerance and Escalation

Tolerance and escalation occur in substance addiction when the addict requires more of a substance or a stronger substance to achieve and maintain the same high that he or she seeks. Tolerance and escalation occur with sexual addiction when the addict spends increasing amounts of time engaging in the addiction or when the intensity level of his/her sexual fantasies and activities increases. Because of tolerance and escalation, many sex addicts eventually find themselves engaging in sexual behaviors that did not even occur to them early in the addictive process. Some behave in ways that defy their personal moral code, spiritual beliefs, and, in some cases, the law. Some progress to viewing illicit or bizarre images, while others simply devote more and more of their energy and valuable time to sex.

Withdrawal

With sexual addiction, withdrawal often manifests emotionally and psychologically rather than physically, as it does with substance abuse (e.g., delirium tremens when detoxing from alcohol). Sex addicts going through withdrawal tend to become depressed or restless, lonely, irritable, and dissatisfied. Withdrawal, like tolerance, is not a required component of a sex addiction diagnosis, but most sex addicts experience it.

Denial

Sex addicts in denial are oblivious to the process, costs, and reality of their addiction. They routinely disregard warning signs that would be obvious to a healthier individual. They frequently blame the consequences of their sexual behavior on other people or situations. In short, they are frequently unable or unwilling to recognize the negative consequences of their sexual behavior until a related crisis knocks on their door.

Throughout the twentieth century, sex addiction professionals tended to place a strong emphasis on committed, monogamous relationships as the ultimate goal of recovery from sexual addiction. However, we have learned over time that marriage and long-term commitments are not required for everyone seeking sexual healing or sobriety (unless one is already in a committed, long-term monogamous relationship). In this present era, healing from sexual addiction can include many different types of meaningful, open, and honest sexual or romantic connections—as long as they are not secretive, abusive to oneself or others, used repeatedly to avoid feelings, or cause problems for the addict and the addict's loved ones.

To summarize, sex addicts do not need to be married to be in sexual recovery. They must, however, be attached to their sexual partners and not treat or use them as objects. In fact, some persons in sexual recovery have been through so much adolescent trauma that they may never be able to create and sustain meaningful monogamy. However, this does not preclude them from healing, recovering, forming meaningful interpersonal connections (sexual and otherwise), and feeling happy and at peace with themselves. In other words, we now see that sexual recovery is more about personal integrity, relationship building that may or may not incorporate sex, and the elimination of impulsive and problematic sexual behavior.

THE CYCLE OF SEXUAL ADDICTION

All addictions are cyclical in nature, with no clear beginning or end and one stage leading to the next (and then the next, and the next, and the next), leaving the addict stuck in an endless, downwardly spiraling loop.

With sexual addiction, various models of the addictive cycle have been proposed, modified, and expanded upon, and there are now many versions, each with merit. I generally prefer and utilize a six-stage model that follows.

Stage 1: Trigger
Stage 2: Fantasy
Stage 3: Ritualization
Stage 4: Acting Out
Stage 5: Numbing
Stage 6: Despair

Stage One: Triggers (Shame/Blame/Guilt/Other Strong Emotions)

Triggers are catalysts that create a need/desire to act out sexually. Most often, triggers are some sort of "pain agent." Pain agents include both emotional/psychological and physical discomfort, either short-term or long-term. Depression, anxiety, loneliness, boredom, stress, shame, anger, and any other uncomfortable feeling can easily trigger a sex addict's desire to escape, avoid, and dissociate. Positive agents can also serve as triggers like the icing on a cake. So if a sex addict gets fired from his or her job, they will want to act out sexually; also, if that same addict gets a great new job, they will want to act out sexually.

Triggers can also be visual (seeing a sexy image on a billboard), auditory (hearing a noise that reminds the addict of sexual activity), olfactory (smelling the perfume of a past sexual partner), or even touch or taste-related. Suppose such triggers are not recognized early and dealt with in a healthy way (dissipated via a healthy, non-addictive coping mechanism like talking to supportive friends, family members, or a therapist). In that case, the cycle inevitably slides forward into stage two.

Stage Two: Fantasy

After being triggered and therefore needing to emotionally escape and dissociate, sex addicts often unconsciously turn to their primary coping mechanism: sexual fantasy. They start thinking about how much they enjoyed past sexual encounters and how much they would enjoy a sexual encounter either right now or in the near future. At this point, the addict is preoccupied to the point of obsession with his or her sexual fantasies. On this day, they might flirt with the grocery clerk that they barely noticed just a day or two prior.

Every person encountered by the addict (both in-person and online) is viewed as a sexual object or simply "in the way." The addict's fantasies do not involve memories of prior bad experiences or related negative consequences. Once the addict's mind is mired in fantasy, it is very difficult to stop the addictive cycle without outside intervention.

Stage Three: Ritualization

Ritualization is where fantasy moves toward reality. This stage adds excitement, intensity, and arousal. For example, the addict logs on to the computer and goes to his or her favorite porn site, or hops in the car and drives to a place where sex workers congregate, or begins the process of booking an out-of-town business trip on which he or she can act out sexually without restraint, or simply opens up their favorite "adult friend finder" app. This stage of the cycle is also known as *the bubble* or *the trance* because the addict is psychologically and emotionally lost to it. Real-world concerns disappear as the addict focuses more and more intently on their sexual fantasies. This stage of the addiction (rather than the sex act itself) evokes the escapist neurochemical high that (sex) addicts seek. As such, sex addicts typically try to stretch this stage out for as long as possible—looking at porn, cruising for casual sex, chatting via webcams, losing hours on a sex app, and the like for many hours (or even days) before moving to the next stage.

Stage Four: Sexual Acting Out

Most non-sex addicts think that this stage is the ulti-mate goal of sexual addiction because this is where actual sex and orgasm takes place (either solo or with others). However, as stated above, the fantasy-fueled escape and dissociation of this stage is the real objective. In fact, many will try to put off actual sex and orgasm for as long as possible because orgasm ends the fantasy-driven escapist high and tosses the addict back into the real world with all of its issues and problems. In other words, sex addicts are seeking more to escape emotional discomfort than to experience the pleasure of orgasm. Orgasm brings their high to an abrupt, screeching halt.

Stage Five: Numbing

After acting out, sex addicts attempt to emotionally distance themselves emotionally from what they've just done. They justify their behaviors, telling themselves, *If my spouse were nicer to me, I wouldn't need to do this.* They minimize their behaviors, telling themselves, Nobody knows that I just spent six hours looking at and masturbating to pornography, and nobody got hurt by what *I did, so it's no big deal.* They rationalize their behaviors, telling themselves, Hooking up with people online for mutual masturbation isn't really cheating because I don't actually touch the other person, and I don't even give that person my real name, etc. In other words, in this stage of the cycle, the addict's denial kicks in full force as a way to temporarily protect him or her from the next stage.

Stage Six: Despair (Shame/Anxiety/Depression)

Eventually, numbing will dissipate for most sex addicts. And when it does, many will start to feel ashamed and remorseful. Exacerbating these unwanted emotions is that they also feel powerless to stop their addiction cycle. Furthermore, whatever reality they were attempting to escape in the first place returns, bringing with it any self-loathing, anxiety, or depression they were already experiencing.

And, as you may recall, this is exactly the sort of emotional discomfort that triggers sexual addiction in the first place. As such, over time, stage six spins the self-perpetuating cycle right back to stage one. Where it starts all over again.

Repeating the Cycle Builds Tolerance AND Trains the Brain

The sexual addiction cycle typically intensifies with each repetition, requiring more of the same behavior or more intense behavior to reach or maintain the same neurochemical high over time. This transforms from a repetitive loop into a downward spiral—one characteristic of all forms of addiction—leading to a relationship, work, health, financial, legal, and other crises. And all of these crises also qualify as emotional triggers, which can set the same process in motion yet again.

How Can the Cycle Be Stopped?

The cycle of sexual addiction is best interrupted in the early portion of stage one when the addict's emotional triggers (the experiences and emotions that activate a desire to sexually act out) first arise. If and when the addict learns to recognize the early signs of emotional discomfort like stress, certain types of imagery, people, situations, places, then he or she can engage in contrary actions designed to:

A: Stop the escalating fantasies before they lead to ritualization and acting out

B: Deal with the unwanted, uncomfortable feelings or triggers in an emotionally healthy way and not act them out

This will be covered in greater depth in subsequent chapters.

Unfortunately, some people may misuse the label "sex addiction" to define virtually any type of sexual behavior that doesn't meet their own moral standards (religious, cultural, personal, etc.).

- She's had two affairs, so she must be a sex addict.
- He has had sex with men. He's obviously a sex addict.
- You can be excommunicated in our church for watching pornography. I've heard he watched porn at least a half-dozen times, so he must be a sex addict. Why else would he take such risks?

Other individuals can misuse the sex addiction label as a catch-all excuse for virtually any type of sexual misconduct. In other words, people who get caught red-handed engaging in inappropriate, problematic, possibly even illegal sexual behavior will sometimes blame their actions on an addiction, hoping to avoid or at least to minimize the judgment and punishment they experience. Occasionally, these individuals are sexually addicted; however, this is not always the case. In either situation, a sexual addiction diagnosis is never meant to justify bad conduct or absolve people of responsibility for their behavior.

Unfortunately, it is not only laypeople's or the media's "diagnoses" that cause problems. There are many well-meaning but misinformed therapists out there who are willing to label anything as sexual addiction.

To a large extent, this is because, surprisingly, the mental health profession in the United States requires very little training in human sexual behavior. As a result, some therapists incorrectly believe that any type of sexual or gender-driven dysphoria (unhappiness, shame, and self-loathing) should be treated as an addiction. This is simply not true. The fact that a person feels bad about sexualized thoughts, feelings, desires, or actions does not imply that they are a sex addict for engaging in them. Yes, that individual *might* be a sex addict, but only if their behavior meets the primary criteria for a sexual addiction diagnosis: ongoing obsession, loss of control, and repeated negative consequences, and all the rest. For clarity, below, I have compiled a list of things that sex addiction is not.

Sex addiction is not fun.

When you say the words sexual addiction, the knee-jerk response is often something like: "Hey, sounds fun. Sign me up." In fact, sex addiction is the polar opposite of fun. It's a compulsion that, like any other form of addiction, leads to guilt, depression, anxiety, and a slew of other negative consequences.

Sex addiction is not an excuse for bad behavior.

As previously stated, many people who are caught engaged in shameful, objectionable (such as an affair) or illegal sexual behavior attempt to use sex addiction as a catch-all excuse in order to escape or at the very least minimize the stigma and punishment they may face.

Sometimes, these individuals are sexually addicted, but just as often, they are not. Either way, a diagnosis of sexual addiction never *justifies* bad behavior. Rather than offering an excuse, a diagnosis of sexual addiction places a responsibility on the person to accept the problem and change their behavior in the future. Sex addicts are never absolved of blame for the issues that their actions have created. In fact, part of healing from sexual addiction is admitting what you've done, accepting any consequences, and making amends as best you can.

Sex addiction is not related to sexual orientation or gender identity.

Neither homosexual, bisexual, nor trans-related arousal patterns are factors in diagnosing sexual addiction, even if those arousal patterns are ego-*dystonic* (unwanted). Being gay, lesbian, bisexual, or transgender does not make you a sex addict any more than being straight makes you a sex addict. Sometimes self-loathing homosexuals, transgender people, or bisexuals will seek out sex addiction treatment, hoping it will change their sexual orientation or identity.

They occasionally do this at the request of a misguided clinician. It is, however, impossible to change one's arousal template. If you like men, that's the way it is; if you like women, it's the same story; and if you like both genders, you'd better get used to it because it's not going to change no matter how much analysis you have or how many twelve-step meetings you attend. Simply put, "sexual addiction is not defined in any way by who or what turns you on."

Sex addiction is not related to fetishes or paraphilias (kink).

Fetishes and paraphilias are recurring, intense, sexually arousing fantasies, urges, and behaviors involving nonhuman objects, specific body parts, one's own or one's sexual partner's suffering, or nonconsensual sex (in appearance or actuality). We're talking about BDSM (a la *Fifty Shades of Grey*), foot worship, chubby chasing, diapers/infantilism, *etc.* Fetishes and paraphilias may cause an individual to keep sexual secrets, feel embarrassed and distress, and even feel out of control, but they do not indicate sexual addiction. In fact, they are pathologized only if they cause significant distress and impairment of social, occupational, or other important areas of functioning to that individual. Even if a fetish or paraphilia qualifies as pathologic (for example, bestiality), it is not the same as sexual addiction. So, once again, sexual addiction is not in any way defined by who or what it is that turns you on. Many people have sexual concerns but are not sex addicts.

Sex addiction is not just a guy thing.

The common perception is that only men are sex addicts. This is not true. Plenty of women are sexually and romantically addicted. That said, men are usually easier to diagnose because they are generally more forthcoming about the purely sexual nature of what they are doing. On the other hand, women tend to talk about sex in terms of relationships, even when they're having just as much sex, and the same types of sex, as their male counterparts.

Sex addiction is not driven by drug use.

Sometimes drug users and drug addicts, particularly those who abuse cocaine, methamphetamine, and other stimulants/party drugs, can become hypersexual when high. This is especially true in men who use Viagra or another erection-enhancing drug. This, however, does not imply that these people are sex addicts. If the hypersexual behavior stops when the drug use stops, a diagnosis of sexual addiction is unlikely.

Sexual addiction is not a symptom of bipolar disorder, ADHD (attention-deficit/hyperactivity disorder), OCD (obsessive-compulsive disorder), or any other psychiatric condition.

To diagnose sexual addiction, professionals must first rule out various major mental health disorders that may include hyper-sexuality or impulsive sexual behavior as a symptom. Active stages of bipolar disorder, obsessive-compulsive disorder, and attention-deficit/hyperactivity disorder are among them. In other words, not everyone who is impulsively or compulsively sexual has a problem driven by sexual addiction; hypersexual and impulsive sexual behaviors are legitimate symptoms of many other disorders. That said, it is certainly possible to have any of the aforementioned psychiatric conditions and be sexually addicted. Much as an alcoholic can also have OCD, *etc.*

Sex addiction is not the same thing as sexual offending.

By definition, sexual offending involves either illegal or non-consensual sexual behavior. This isn't the same thing as sexual addiction. Yes, the behavior of approximately 10 percent of all sex addicts may escalate into offending—most often engaging in lower-level offenses like voyeurism, exhibitionism, viewing inappropriate pornography, and engaging in prostitution. Nevertheless, sexual offending is not indicative of sexual addiction. It is critically important that the criteria for sex addiction be very strictly applied when dealing with sex offenders, as these individuals are the group most likely to self-identify as sex addicts in an attempt to avoid judgment or punishment.

Sex addiction therapy is sex-positive!

Some people are worried that sex addiction therapists are attempting to become the new "sex police," imposing moral, cultural, or religious values on sexuality and creating a narrow version of sexual health. Sadly, this fear is not entirely unfounded. There are indeed some moralist or highly religiously driven therapists who misuse and misapply the sex addiction diagnosis, using it to marginalize and pathologize sexual behaviors that don't mesh with their personal or religious belief systems. Homosexuality, bisexuality, transgenderism, recreational porn use, casual sex, polyamory, and fetishes—all of which today fall within the spectrum of normal and healthy adult sexuality—have at times been misdiagnosed as sexual addiction.

In reality, as stated previously, sexual addiction has nothing whatsoever to do with who or what it is that turns a person on. Instead, as described throughout this book, sex addiction is about using the excitement and intensity of sexual fantasies and behaviors (of whatever kind) to emotionally numb out by evoking emotional arousal, excitement, and fantasy-fueled distraction.

SEX ADDICTION—THE BASICS: TRIGGERS, ESCALATION, AND DENIAL

Regardless of the addiction, be it substance or behavioral, there are three underlying components that most often drive and perpetuate the problem: triggers, escalation, and denial. Because they are so important and so pervasive in all forms of addiction, including sexual addiction, those two topics are addressed more fully in this section, along with addiction's third underlying element, denial. Before addressing these three topics, however, it is useful to have a solid understanding of what addiction does to the human brain.

The Neurobiology of Addiction

One of the most common questions faced by sex addicts and their loved ones is: why is it so difficult to simply stop? Answering this question helps to understand how addiction affects the human brain. Essentially, in a normal, healthy (non-addicted) brain, our naturally occurring "pleasure" or "rewards center"—registers pleasurable feelings in response to naturally occurring, life-affirming behaviors such as eating, helping others, joining with our community, being sexual, etc. These activities are rewarded because they (feel good) also ensure the survival of both the individual and the human species. This is intelligent design (or evolution) at its finest.

These sensations of pleasure result from the release of various neurochemicals, primarily dopamine, along with adrenaline, serotonin, oxytocin, and a few others.

When pleasure is experienced in the brain's rewards center, other portions of the brain are alerted, most notably those involving mood, memory, and decision-making. Basically, the rewards center tells the mood, memory, and decision-making regions how much it enjoyed eating, helping, having sex, etc. In this way, we learn which activities are pleasurable. Over time, we associate these behaviors with enjoyment and a sense of well-being, and we make future decisions based on this information.

Unfortunately, our rewards center can be tampered with as well. Alcohol, addictive medications, and compulsive habits of highly stimulating behaviors (sex, romance, gambling, spending, video gaming, etc.) are just a few examples and can be abused to artificially stimulate the system, flooding the brain with unusually high levels of dopamine—anywhere from two to hundreds of times the amount provided by the normal pleasurable activity. That's quite a jolt of pleasure juice! This enjoyment-related knowledge is transmitted to areas of the brain that deal with decision-making, memory, and mood just as it is with other pleasurable experiences. Is it any surprise, then, that we want more, more, and more things that feel, taste, sound, and smell good? (Think sex, chocolate, winning, approval, etc.)

To make things worse, our brains are designed to respond to the information we get. The brain responds to excessive dopamine levels over time by generating less and less dopamine or removing dopamine receptors as addictive inputs are continuously engaged (through repeated substance use, gambling, sex, or whatever). (When dopamine "plugs in" to a dopamine receptor, it causes pleasure.) To put it another way, as addiction develops, the brain is programmed to anticipate artificially high levels of dopamine (pleasure). In this way, loving an addictive substance or behavior will turn into wanting/needing it, and then desire takes over, implying that you must have it. Addicts want/need to continue using despite the fact that the addictive stimulation (drugs, alcohol, sex, romance, gambling, etc.) no longer offers the same degree of pleasure. This is where triggers, escalation, and denial come into play.

Understanding Triggers

Triggers are the thoughts, experiences, and feelings that induce a strong desire—the craving—to ingest an addictive substance or engage in addictive behavior. When addictive cravings set in, it is very difficult to stop the ensuing addiction cycle. This is why addicts sometimes find it hard to remain sober, despite their best efforts.

Unfortunately, anything that triggers the brain to remember the long-lost pleasure of addiction is a potential precursor for cravings and relapse.

Internal triggers: These are typically emotional (or sometimes physical) discomforts of any kind—depression, shame, anxiety, anger, fear, guilt, remorse, boredom, and so on. For example, if/when a married sex addict's spouse is away for a few days (or even a few hours), he or she may feel lonely, which may trigger a desire to act out sexually.

External triggers: These can be people, places, things, or events. For example, if a sex addict sees an old partner with whom he or she once had sex, he or she may be triggered to act out sexually. Addicts must also deal with intertwined triggers (both external and internal). For instance, if/when a sex addict argues with his or her spouse or has a bad day at work (an external trigger), he or she is likely to experience emotional discomfort, say frustration or anger (internal triggers), with both triggers leading to a desire to sexually act out. And visual triggers that remind the addict of his or her addiction may exacerbate this desire (such as driving past strip clubs, prostitutes, and drug dealers).

Surprisingly, not all triggers are bad. Material success and positive emotions can sometimes elicit a desire to celebrate, and thus a desire to drink, use drugs, act out sexually, gamble, spend, and so on. Some of the more common internal causes for sexual acting-out include:

- Any unmet need for validation and affection
- Unresolved resentments and anger
- Loneliness
- Boredom
- Fear
- Anxiety
- Frustration
- Low self-esteem
- Shame (feeling useless, worthless, or unlovable)
- Stress
- Feeling unappreciated
- Sadness or grief

Some of the more common external causes for sexual acting-out include:

- Unstructured time alone
- Travel (especially alone)
- Relationship breakups, changes, and losses
- Unexpected life changes (job, finances, etc.)
- Unexpected losses or tragedies
- Highly stimulating positive experiences (having a baby, getting promoted)

- Drug or alcohol use
- Arguments
- Reprimands
- Financial insecurity
- Family strife (for example, a child struggling in school)
- An emotionally or physically unavailable spouse

Both of the preceding lists could be expanded indefinitely because each person's triggers are unique to them. Even memories of past traumas can act as triggers in the present. For instance, if my boss speaks to one of my coworkers crossly, this might remind me of my alcoholic raging father, which brings up a slew of emotional discomfort—fear, anger, shame, etc. —and I, therefore, am triggered, even though my boss's tone has nothing at all to do with me in the present moment.

Unfortunately, triggers are unavoidable but not so how we can learn to monitor and deal with them. Consider alcoholics driving past billboard advertisements for beer, scotch, and vodka. Consider drug addicts who watch television crime dramas in which people sell or use drugs. Think about all of the attractive people (potential sexual partners) a sex addict comes into contact with regularly, both online and in person.

Then the roller coaster of life and the emotions that even an average day can induce. Triggers are everywhere, and addicts can do nothing about it except learn to recognize and deal with them in healthy ways (a process discussed in detail in later chapters). For now, I will simply say that if an addict can learn to identify his or her triggers and stop them in their tracks—before they induce undue craving—then he or she has a much better chance to stay sober.

Understanding Escalation

Addicts of all types typically experience an increasing tolerance to the mood-altering effects of a pleasurable addictive substance or behavior. (Remember, the brain adjusts to excessive dopamine levels caused by continued use of addictive substances and behaviors by producing less dopamine and reducing the number of dopamine receptors in the brain.) As a result, addicts must, over time, use more of an addictive substance/behavior or a more intense substance/behavior to achieve and maintain the desired neurochemical high. Janet, in the example above, did both.

Consider drug addiction if you're having trouble understanding this. Almost no one starts shooting heroin right away. Instead, drug addicts begin by smoking marijuana or abusing prescription medications. Their tolerance grows over time, and as a result, their habits become more severe. Maybe they start smoking marijuana all the time, or maybe they start popping pills by the handful. Eventually, as their brain adapts, even that level of usage does not get or keep them high as they would like. Many will eventually "graduate" to drugs like cocaine, methamphetamine, and heroin, abusing these stronger substances to get high (the way they used to). At first, they may simply mix a small amount of cocaine or meth into a joint or cigarette or mix a small amount of heroin into the pills they've learned to crush and snort (for faster effect). Finally, without having made a conscious decision to do so, they "find themselves" cooking and injecting their new drug of choice.

Sex addicts' behavior escalates in a similar way. For example, many people regard viewing and masturbating to generic (so-called "vanilla") online porn as an enjoyable and relatively innocuous occasional activity akin to drinking a few beers. However, for some people, what begins as a harmless recreation can become an all-consuming activity, pushing the user away from relationships, family, work, hobbies, and other life-affirming activities. Hours, even days, are lost to sexual fantasy. Over time, the user may find that they are looking at and being turned on by increasingly more intense sexual imagery and extending their use into other sexual activities (webcam sex, casual sex, anonymous sex, and the like).

Common forms of escalation that occur with sexual addiction include (but are not even remotely limited to) the following:

- Serial affairs or multiple affairs at the same time
- High numbers of casual and anonymous sexual encounters
- Hours, sometimes even days lost to pornography or other forms of online sexual behavior
- Alcohol or drug abuse concurrent with sexual addiction
- Unsafe sex
- Sex with strangers or dangerous people
- Sex in dangerous locations

- Sensual massage, escorts, and prostitution (buying or selling)
- Viewing illicit or unusual (for the addict) imagery
- Exhibitionism (either online or in person)
- Voyeurism (either online or in person)

For many sex addicts, escalation can involve a cross or co-occurring addiction. These coexisting addictive disorders are discussed in a later chapter. For now, let's just say that sex addicts' most common secondary addiction is to stimulant drugs like cocaine or methamphetamine. These drugs cause feelings of euphoria, intensity, and power, along with the drive to obsessively do whatever activity the user wishes to engage in, including having sex, for extended periods. Some users say that meth, for instance, allows them to be sexual for an entire day, even two or three days, without sleeping, eating, or coming down—especially if an erection-enhancing drug like Viagra, Levitra, or Cialis is along for the ride.

Sometimes meth is blatantly advertised on hookup and escort websites and apps: "Come over for PNP with me and my friend Tina." ("PNP" is shorthand for "party and play," indicating the person who posted this is seeking both sex and drug use, and "Tina" is one of many common street names for meth.)

Understanding Denial

Active sex addicts rarely blame their unhappiness and life challenges on their escapist sexual fantasies and behaviors. Even when they are neck-deep in consequences, they do not consider their sexual acting out to be a contributing factor. In fact, they frequently see their behavior as the solution rather than the cause of their emotional distress and other life issues. This is the face of denial. Put simply, sex addicts are nearly always out of touch with the costs of their addictive sexual behavior, at least until a major crisis hits. Before that, they ignore blatant warning signs, destroy relationships, breeze past workplace reprimands as well as related drug abuse, STDs (sexually transmitted diseases), unwanted pregnancies, financial problems, etc.

They simply refuse to see or cannot see the destructive effects of their sexual fantasies and behavior. Again, this is denial. Put simply, unlike healthy individuals, use past mistakes as a guide to future decision making, while addicts choose to ignore past problems that are related to their addictive behavior. In short, they place their compulsive search for sexual intensity at the top of their priority list without a second thought, no matter the cost. Instead of heeding the many warning signs of a serious problem, they rationalize, minimize, and justify their behavior, frequently blaming others for the consequences they face. For instance:

- If the police had been out chasing real criminals, I wouldn't have gotten caught up in that prostitution sting.
- If my wife weren't such a cold fish, I wouldn't need to look at porn, and then I wouldn't have been fired from my job for misusing company equipment.
- If my husband hadn't gained so much weight, I

wouldn't have lost interest in him and had so
many affairs, and we wouldn't be divorced now.

For some sex addicts, denial is so deep that they somehow manage to stay blissfully unaware of the nature and extent of their problematic sexual behaviors, even when those behaviors escalate to ruining their relationships and lives. In short, they find ways to ignore the seriousness of their actions so they can continue with those actions, most often by blaming their poor decisions on someone or something outside of themselves. Denial for active addicts means externalizing the blame for their problems by making them someone or something else's fault. And this willful ignorance can go on for years. In fact, when confronted in the early stages of treatment with an adult-life sex and relationship history, many sex addicts are shocked to finally "discover" the extent and depth of their addictive behaviors.

Denial and Addiction

Denial is characterized by a complex series of internal lies and deceptions. Typically, each fabrication is backed up by one or more rationalizations, with each rationalization bolstered by even more lies. When viewed objectively, denial is about as structurally sound like a house of cards in a stiff breeze, but active addicts act and frequently feel as if they live in an impenetrable bomb shelter. They zealously defend their flimsy lies and deceptions, no matter how ridiculous they are. In time, they start to believe their lies, and they expect others to do so as well. And because addicts buy into their dishonesty, their behaviors, no matter how crazy, can seem utterly reasonable to them.

Yes, the rest of the world may easily see through the smokescreen, but addicts cannot (or will not). Instead, they remain mired in the murky muck of their denial until their functional world devolves into a mess of addiction-related consequences.

Addicts never intend to destroy their relationships, hurt loved ones, ignore their children, ruin their careers, wreck their finances, get arrested, or do anything else. Nonetheless, they frequently find themselves in these situations, progressing gradually as their denial worsens. They become less able (and less willing) to see the link between their increasing personal problems and their escalating addictive behaviors as time passes.

Deaf to the complaints, concerns, and criticisms of those around them—even those they claim to love—they will devalue and dismiss (or blame) those who attempt to point out the problem.

Instead of accepting that they may have a serious problem, they dismiss attempts to help them and accuse others of nagging, being prudish and restrictive, not understanding them, or expecting too much of them. They do this not because they don't care but because they "need" to protect their addiction and are embarrassed.

TYPES OF SEXUAL ADDICTION

Not every sex addict experiences the same form of sexual addiction. Some behaviors common to many sex addicts do not begin as early but develop over time. Such behaviors may range from the seemingly normal sexual encounter with another consenting adult to illegal and abusive behavior, such as rape or incest. The behaviors described here, particularly sexually abusive behaviors, reflect deeper levels of emotional pathology.

SEX WITH A CONSENTING PARTNER

Let's look at this with a few examples. Mary has had sex with at least five hundred men. At any one time, she has ongoing relationships with eight men, and on a given day, she may have sex with three or four of them. At night, she frequents bars to recruit new partners. Looking for the love she never found in her father, she escapes her depression through frequent sexual encounters.

Mary is a sex addict who engages in frequent sex with

many consenting partners. Other sex addicts may have only one affair every few years. Still, other sex addicts have sex with only one partner, and sex happens infrequently. This kind of sexual activity occurs between both heterosexuals and homosexuals.

Some persons mistakenly equate sexual addiction with homosexuality. They think acting out in homosexual ways is equivalent to addiction. However, this is not the case. Many homosexuals are not addicted to sexual activity. Some live celibate or monogamous lives with a committed partner. The source of the confusion could be that many contributing factors leading to sexual addiction may also lead to homosexuality. There is very little research on this, but I offer two observations based on my experience. First, since addiction and homosexuality may share some causative factors, there could be a higher percentage of homosexuals who are sexually addicted. Second, homosexual men are more likely to be addicted than homosexual women.

Sexual addiction with a consenting partner can be placed along a continuum. At one end are those who have only one partner and engage in sex infrequently. At the other end are those who have many partners and engage in sex frequently. Between are varying numbers of partners and frequencies. The definition of sexual addiction does not depend on the number of partners but on why addicts practice sexual behavior and whether they can stop the behavior. Therefore, even if a person has had only one affair, it could have been addictive if sex was used to escape feelings, was not an expression of intimacy between two people, and led to destructive consequences.

For some sex addicts, the consenting partner is the spouse. Some married couples avoid talking to each other by engaging in multiple daily sexual acts. A husband may ask his wife to perform sexual activities she doesn't like and is even repulsed by. Spousal consent to these activities may be a sign of sexual co-addiction.

CYBER-SEX

The growth of sexual relationships between consenting adults on the Internet is often referred to as cyber-sex. Let's examine Cyber-sex with a few examples.

Betty, a pastor's wife, first started participating in Internet chat rooms; she became so engrossed in her online relationships she lost all track of time. She didn't know what month it was and could not recall what she had done with her family, at work, or church. She experienced a virtual blackout. She was so intoxicated with fantasy, lust, and excitement that her mind went numb. Within the second month of online usage, she progressed from chat to sexual chat, to phone sex, to meeting three men for sex.

George, a mild-mannered farmer, loved to play online games. He often asked for a female partner. Sometimes this led to casual chatting after the game, but other times it led to sexual talk and, in one instance, meeting a woman in person for sex.

Mary, a businesswoman, traveled to many cities for her job. Before she left on every trip, she arranged to meet with men she found through online "connecting" services. She was active in ongoing affairs with three men in three different cities.

These three stories illustrate the prevalence of online sexual connecting. In each case, the people involved were otherwise socially inhibited. They would not have been comfortable meeting people in public. They would have been even less comfortable making sexual connections face-to-face. However, the relative ease of connecting anonymously through a computer ultimately gave them the courage to connect in person.

For some, online sexual connecting may never go beyond sex chatting, but it can progress to actual sexual experience for others. The number of services that connect people to sexual activity has increased dramatically. One service advertises itself as an "adult friend finder." This is especially appealing because every addict struggles with loneliness. We all have deep desires to be in a community, to belong, and to be included. The Internet gives shy and otherwise timid people a way to make relational connections. This doorway originally appeals to loneliness and legitimate desires for connection but can easily progress to sexual activity and eventually to addiction.

PROSTITUTION

The use of prostitution is very common for many sex addicts. Because prostitution clients pay for sex as if it were a business transaction, they do not need to get involved with their partners like they might have to if they began an affair. Some addicts even justify prostitution by saying,

"No one gets hurt."

Today we have massage parlors, escort services, and "modeling" agencies to go along with the traditional hookers on the street. For the right price, prostitutes will even come to a client's home. Adult bookstores and bars feature various forms of nude dancing, and often the dancers or models engage in prostitution.

One popular form of prostitution is actually legal and takes place over the telephone. Late-night television is peppered with commercials for numbers that enable callers to "discuss" various sexual activities. The ads appeal to both erotic and emotional needs by featuring attractive women who talk about loneliness, friendship, connection, and intimacy.

Sex addicts spend small fortunes on prostitution, just like alcoholics who drink away their paychecks. At our hospital, we treat sex addicts who have spent thousands of dollars on these phone services.

Prostitution is increasingly available on the Internet via chat rooms, downloadable images and video, and other forms of "virtual reality." Many prostitutes who used to need a pimp, escort service, or massage parlor to find clients can now do so independently using the Internet.

Anyone can create a website and market illicit services online. The same Triple-A Engine that makes Internet pornography so powerful—accessible, affordable, anonymous—also makes online prostitution powerful.

Prostitution appeals to the fantasizing nature of the sex addict. In the movie Pretty Woman, for example, when the businessman portrayed by Richard Gere asks the prostitute portrayed by Julia Roberts what her name is, she replies, "What would you like it to be?" She knows many of her customers have elaborate fantasies about whom or what they want her to be. Prostitution reinforces the fantasizing mindset of the sex addict.

Sex addicts may experience more kindness and nurture from a prostitute than anyone else. One sex addict loves to be treated like a baby by prostitutes. He gets powdered, diapered, and cooed over as if he were an infant. With sex addicts and prostitution, we are not just dealing with perverted adults looking to satisfy their lust. We are dealing with babies and young children in adult bodies who are looking for love in all the wrong places.

EXHIBITIONISM AND VOYEURISM

Exhibitionism and voyeurism are less common than other forms of sexual addiction but still destructive. Both behaviors can be illegal, and those who are caught may be arrested. The stereotypes of exhibitionism and voyeurism are the "flasher" in a raincoat or the "Peeping Tom" lurking outside a window. However, these addictions are complicated and express themselves in many ways.

Mary, for example, owned a transparent green blouse that left little to the imagination. She wore it to various bars, not so much to recruit new partners to watch the reactions of men who saw her. Arousing them gave her a sense of control she never had when her father and brothers sexually molested her.

Jay loved to go into clothing stores with dressing rooms in the middle of the store. He took clothes in them he never intended to buy and left the door slightly open, waiting for women to come by. When he saw their surprised expressions, he felt a rush of excitement. Jay was addicted to his fantasies of those looks and what they might mean. He was also addicted to the adrenaline rush.

Tom, another sex addict, also liked to frequent clothing stores. He loitered in sections that sold women's underwear, pretending to buy something for his wife. Tom stationed himself close to the dressing rooms hoping to catch a glimpse of someone changing.

These are only a few of the many and varied ways that sex addicts can express themselves. Browsing in lingerie departments, positioning oneself to get a look when someone bends over, or simply undressing someone with the eyes are forms of voyeurism.

In addition to physical exposure and voyeurism, a person can perform these activities emotionally. Some addicts tell sexual jokes to get a sexual high. Other addicts are turned on by hearing intimate details of sexual activity. Such addicts may, in turn, talk about their own sex lives, thereby exhibiting themselves emotionally. This form of sexual addiction is often found in the counseling and clergy professions, where it is easy to gain access to the intimate details of people's lives. Not only is this a violation of professional ethics, but it can also be extremely uncomfortable for the counselee.

INDECENT LIBERTIES

Indecent liberties occur when a person initiates physical contact with another person for sexual excitement. The other person has not agreed to the contact and may even be unaware it happened. Grabbing, pinching, tickling, rubbing up against, and other forms of contact in places such as elevators and grocery stores may constitute indecent liberty.

The word groping can apply to this kind of activity. Clinically, it is often referred to as frateurism. Even hugs as an expression of caring may have a sexual meaning to the sex addict.

An individual referred to himself as the "hugging priest." Almost all his female friends complained about how uncomfortable they felt with his hugs. Another individual loved to get on crowded buses and rub up against women there. He often touched these women in sexual ways as well. Even the awareness that he might get slapped gave him a sense of excitement.

This form of sexual addiction reveals the deep needs we all have to touch and be touched. When the natural desire is confused with sexual lust, it can lead to this abusive behavior.

OBSCENE PHONE CALLS

Obscene phone calls aren't limited to talking dirty or breathing heavily on the phone. Andrew, for example, was a pastor who called female members of his congregation to talk about church business and masturbated to the sound of their voices. Another pastor randomly called women out of the phone book and tried to arrange meetings, some of which became sexual.

BESTIALITY

Bestiality, or sexual activity with animals, is another broad category and may involve various acts. Bestiality is a problem in some rural cultures where it may even be perceived as a humorous adolescent rite of passage. However, bestiality is certainly not limited to rural areas, and there are pornographic materials devoted specifically to this behavior.

For example, Larry was a New York City policeman who moonlit for a local veterinarian to satisfy his addiction of having sex with large dogs.

This kind of behavior is among the most disgusting and revolting. It shocks our sensibilities because we can't imagine how humans could allow themselves to become involved with animals. The abusive nature of this behavior is obvious. As appalling as this behavior is, if we remember that the sex addict is searching for love, touch, and nurture, it becomes somewhat easier to understand. Animals, like dogs, love to be touched, are always glad to see us coming, and always sad to see us go.

Many of us understand how important pets can be in the lives of otherwise lonely people. Bestiality is another example of how legitimate desires become destructive when they are confused with sexuality.

RAPE, INCEST, AND CHILD MOLESTATION

Some sexual activities are exploitative, abusive, and criminal. Rape, incest, and child molestation are three. Rape occurs when physical force is used to engage a person in sex against their will. Incest is sexual activity between members of a biological family. Child molestation is an adult engaging in sex with a child who is dependent on that adult for care, supervision, or instruction. The adult may use physical force, even if this is limited to the size differential between the adult and the child. The adult may also use emotional force, the authority of the adult's role in that child's life. These forms of sexual activity have serious legal consequences and generally involve prison sentences.

The term *pedophile* is often used to describe an adult sexually attracted to children under the age of twelve. Sex addicts who act out with children are not all pedophiles, and pedophiles are not all sex addicts who act out with children.

Pedophiles may not act on their pathological orientation in addictive ways. Sex addicts who act out with children may not be primarily oriented to children. Many people who act out with children are repeating experiences they had as children. In fact, most sex addicts are victims of childhood sexual abuse. Now that they are adults, they can be in control. This gives them a misguided sense that they have reversed the pain of what happened to them.

Adults who offend in this manner may also be repeating their childhood abuse because it reunites them to the first time their sexual consciousness was aroused. This is known as *imprinting*. When adults continue to act out what was imprinted on them as children, they may be reverting to their childhood feelings of sexual arousal. The concept of imprinting is an important one for anyone who works with adolescents and teens. Having sexual experiences before marriage has potent and long-lasting effects. One's first sexual experience is very powerful and should be reserved for marriage. When this kind of repetition occurs, it perpetuates the cycle of sexual abuse.

In addition to rape, incest, and child molestation, abuse of authority is another exploitive and criminal sexual activity. This includes sexual activity between two adults, not biologically related. One of them is in a position of greater power or authority, such as a doctor, lawyer, teacher, employer, or older adult. This is sometimes referred to as "authority rape." Although the person not in power may have consented to or even initiated the sexual activity, the consent or the initiation is not freely given because the situation is inequitable when one person has greater influence or emotional power over the other. In these situations, the person not in power is the victim.

Authority rape assumes that the victim believes the exploiter to be powerful, knowledgeable, or even "sacred." The victim wants to be part of that power, be nurtured by the authority figure, and do anything to secure this nurturance. The victim may have been molested as a child and now associates sexual activity with nurture. In such cases, the victim projects parent-like qualities to the powerful person.

Some of these criminal forms of activity may reflect sexual addiction, and some may not. Some sex offenders are sociopaths (they have no sense of right and wrong), and they have other personality disorders. For them, acting out sexually may be expressions of these disorders, anger and rage, or a need to punish and control.

This chapter explored several activities a sex addict may engage in; however, this list is by no means complete, and some extreme behaviors may not be discussed.

The most common behaviors are still the building-block behaviors of fantasy, pornography, and masturbation, and some addicts focus on these activities alone. Others who commit more serious forms of sexual addiction may also practice these basic addictive behaviors to control more severe behaviors.

In diagnosing sexual addiction, it is important to consider more than the behaviors alone. It's easy to be distracted by the immoral, illegal, or bizarre nature of some of them. Sex addicts may excuse their addiction to fantasy or pornography by saying, "I've never raped anyone, so I'm not a sex addict." However, if this person engages in any uncontrollable, repetitive sexual behavior, he or she is a sex addict.

Whether sex addicts have committed rape or only fantasized about sex, they have certain traits common to all sex addicts. The next chapter describes these common characteristics.

❊ 3 ❊

CHARACTERISTICS OF SEXUAL ADDICTION

Let's begin this chapter with an example. Bryan is a successful doctor and a respected family man. His bedside manner is quick and terse, but he smiles often and says the right things. A popular man, he has countless friends. But Ryan and his wife generally don't have time for each other, being too distracted by their work, social life, and children.

Lately, after busy days at the hospital, Bryan has been engaging in sex with prostitutes. He also suffers from occasional outbursts of anger at work, but the staff excuses his behavior, saying he is a busy man and the stress of caring for his patients must be great. Everyone around him assumes that since Bryan helps others with their problems, he doesn't have problems himself. They also assume that since people around Bryan like him, Bryan must like himself. But Bryan hates himself, his behaviors, and his work. Being a doctor helps him feel important temporarily, but the feeling wears off. He is beginning to consider suicide.

Fortunately, as strange as it may sound, the chief of staff at Bryan's hospital intervenes. A hospital nurse driving home had witnessed Bryan picking up a prostitute. Bryan is let go from the hospital but offered the opportunity to seek treatment for his problem.

Bryan's story illustrates several characteristics of sexual addiction. It also reflects the cycle of behaviors sex addicts get involved in and the possible consequences that can result. This chapter reviews the characteristics, symptoms, cycle, and consequences of sexual addiction.

POOR SELF-IMAGE

Sex addicts like Bryan have a poor self-image. They perceive themselves as bad, evil people. However, those around them may not know this because sex addicts can act with bravado, be boastful, promote themselves, or appear self-righteous. They may also seem arrogant or obnoxious. Sex addicts who try to convince others of how wonderful they are actually trying to convince themselves that they are good people.

Some sex addicts play a martyr role. Their perception that they are bad leads them to believe that the world and everyone in it doesn't like them and that bad things will always happen. They may feel everyone is trying to take advantage of them, and the only attention they can get is sympathy from those who feel sorry for them. Their behavior is extremely frustrating to relatives and friends because they are never happy, won't take or implement constructive advice, and continue to complain even in the face of apparent success.

Other sex addicts compensate for poor self-image by overachieving. They think if they receive praise for their achievements, they will feel better about themselves. However, whatever they might accomplish in life is never good enough to convince them that they are good people.

Always looking for the next triumph or accomplishment, they become addicted to the high of winning. Some sexually addicted pastors are addicted to praise and admiration. But the temporary fix of being complimented on a sermon doesn't last long. By Sunday afternoon, the old convictions of innate badness return.

Still, others may be underachievers, never quite living up to their potential. They believe they will never amount to anything and are afraid to risk trying for fear of failure. They would rather live with the possibility they could accomplish something if they did try. "If I had wanted to, I could have gone to law school and become a lawyer, but it just didn't work out," they may say.

Sex addicts may seem very self-sufficient. A basic belief is that no one will take care of them because no one loves them as they are. At other times or to other people, they may seem very needy as if they always depend on someone else to take care of them.

The negative self-image of the sex addict leads to chronic depression. The vast majority may even think of suicide. Many have tried; some have been successful.

MOOD ALTERATION AND ESCAPE

Larry has a hard time sleeping at night. His job is stressful. His children are rebellious. He worries about money, and he and his wife argue continually about the checkbook and the charge cards. He frequently sneaks off to the bathroom, at home, and at work to masturbate. Now it seems he can't go to sleep without sex. Since his wife is unwilling most of the time, he either fantasizes or masturbates.

Very early in the life of most sex addicts, sex became a solution to painful situations. The pleasurable feelings of sexuality were perhaps the only relief they knew. Sex became an escape, a way of altering their mood. They felt no one else was doing anything for them, so they took matters into their own hands. Sex was a way of coping.

As sex addicts grow up, sex remains a means of coping with stress. When painful feelings occur, sex becomes a way to medicate that pain. Without a more direct form of sexual contact, even fantasy can be soothing to a sex addict.

SENSE OF ENTITLEMENT

When there isn't stress, sex can also be seen as a reward. Since sex addicts believe no one will take care of them and they must do everything for themselves, they begin to build up resentment. While one part of them feels they don't deserve anything and that they are bad people, a deeper and unconscious part of them wants to believe differently. Perhaps this is their spiritual side, the knowledge of their potential for goodness, a connection to a God who loves them.

Sex addicts, however, don't have a healthy sense of how to reward themselves or how to give themselves affirmation. Their anger and resentment are expressed as a sense of entitlement. "I deserve something," they reason. After surviving stressful events, performing well, or doing a good job, sex addicts may believe they deserve to be rewarded sexually.

Perhaps, for example, a sex addict is surviving a bad marriage or a bad job. They stay with it, believing this is the moral and faithful thing to do. However, they also develop the feeling that they need to reward themselves to survive, which medicates their feelings of loneliness and isolation. Sex becomes their reward. A sense of entitlement gives sex addicts the belief that they are justified in their sexual behaviors.

UNMANAGEABILITY AND EFFORTS TO CONTROL

Let's examine the story of an addict who was addicted to pornography. This person was a very religious man who read the Bible continually. He tried various methods to stop pornography addiction, but without success. Finally, he took a biblical injunction seriously and plucked out both eyes because they continued to offend him. This story exemplifies how desperate addicts become in their attempts to control sexual behaviors and how unmanageable these efforts become.

Sex addicts try to stop but can't. They make promises to themselves and employ various strategies to stop the behavior, much like an alcoholic. Some even injure their genitals or other body parts to prevent their behaviors. Some turn rigidly and desperately to religion to stop their behavior. One man was baptized in four different churches to take away his sexual desire.

Usually, this religious approach leads to frustration, shame, and despair. A sex addict believes, "I was bad before. Not even faith can save me; therefore, I must really be a bad person." Often these people turn away from religion altogether. Going to church reminds them of their failure, or they feel God has not loved them enough to take away their lust.

When sex addicts try desperately to control their disease, they may succeed for various time periods. We call this "acting in," "white-knuckling," and more recently, "sexual anorexia." Acting in is the opposite of acting out. This is an extremely significant phenomenon.

Many sex addicts deny they are addicted because they have been acting in or white-knuckling for long periods. In this form of total self-denial, they completely turn off their sexuality. Some married sex addicts may act out with themselves or others but not engage in sexuality with their spouse.

If we believe sex is sacred and a very normal experience between husbands and wives, sexual anorexia is not acceptable. It denies a spouse the God-given gift of sexuality. It might be tempting to believe that those who don't engage in sex at all are living a righteous and pure life. This way of thinking is based on the mistaken belief that the more you deny the body, the more spiritual you become.

Acting in may be based on the Christian's fear of God. It is certainly biblical that we fear God in the same sense we fear parents who love us. We acknowledge their authority and know that, in love, they will punish us if needed to get us back on the right path. Although we may not understand it at the time, punishment is for our correction and rehabilitation.

Christian sex addicts may fear God but not because they believe in God's loving correction. They are simply afraid. Acting in may be their way of manipulating God, so he will not punish them. They turn off sexual feelings not to honor God out of healthy fear but out of an unhealthy fear that God is an angry God.

This phenomenon has many parallels with eating disorders. Anorexics act in refusing to eat in an effort to control their weight, body image, and even their sexuality.

This is crucial for Christians to understand since sexual anorexics often use Christian values to justify their conduct. They mistakenly separate spirit and body in the belief that the body is innately bad. They reason that if the spirit can be "freed" from the desires and temptations of the body, a person will be more acceptable to God.

DENIAL AND DELUSIONS

Some sex addicts have never tried to get help or else have stopped trying. Fear of strong moral judgment or social consequences keeps them silent and alone. They think, "Whom do I tell? Other people will get angry with me, reject me, or go running and screaming out of the room.

I will lose my job, my family, my social standing." These fears create a deep need to be silent and an even more desperate need to control the behavior. This fear of negative consequences and rejection, and the resulting need to control, becomes intense for any addict. If they are ever confronted with their behaviors, they will either deny those behaviors or claim they are in control: "If I wanted to, I could quit."

Often addicts try to justify their behaviors. "I was lonely. My spouse is never sexual with me. People are always taking advantage of me. He seduced me in a weak moment." At other times addicts lie. "I really didn't do that. Where did you get that information? You are wrong. Are you trying to hurt me?"

One of the denial tools is delusion, the belief that the addictive behavior is not really that bad or harmful. It is hard for an outsider to imagine how convincing sex addicts can be to themselves. We might wonder how a person could commit sinful, immoral, and illegal behaviors.

The answer is that they may have deluded themselves into thinking their behaviors aren't that bad and that they really aren't hurting themselves or anyone else.

People who are in denial or deluded may very well benefit from being confronted with their behaviors. Some may also need to suffer the consequences of their behavior to understand their negative and destructive nature.

TOLERANCE

The alcoholic builds alcohol tolerance and therefore needs more and more alcohol to achieve the same mood-altering effect. A sex addict is no different, needing to act out more frequently to obtain the same high.

Hilary frequented relatively safe gay bars in respectable neighborhoods. He made anonymous contacts with men who were gentle like him. This routine became boring, so he began to visit unsafe neighborhoods, where he found rougher men. These encounters became more physically dangerous. While he was afraid of this, it also excited him.

Part of the addictive quality of sex is that it is exciting, sometimes because it is dangerous. When an activity becomes routine, a sex addict may progress to more dangerous or exciting forms of it. This can be as easy as transitioning from private to public masturbation, from having affairs with single people to having affairs with married people, or from finding partners in relatively safe places to finding partners in more risky places. For some, it may also mean progression to illegal forms of sex, such as those described in the previous chapter.

BLACKOUTS

Jerry met a man at a bar. Even though he had wanted to watch the World Series at the bar, he went home with this man and engaged in sex with him. Later that evening, when he left, he was surprised to hear sirens and see crowds of people on the street. Many lights were out, and chaos reigned. While he had been having sex, San Francisco had experienced one of its most devastating earthquakes, yet he had not felt even the most violent of the tremors. Jerry is a good example of how powerful blackouts can be. The state of numbness, and what is clinically called "dissociation," means a person is unaware of even the most violent realities.

Alcohol often causes blackouts—the inability to remember what happened. Alcoholics can wake up in unfamiliar places and not know how they got there or what happened the night before. Sex addicts also experience blackouts when they are intensely involved in what they are doing. They, too, will wake up in strange beds and not know how they got there.

Blackouts occur for several reasons. Many sex addicts use alcohol, and that causes the blackout. Sometimes the experiences are so emotionally painful, the sex addict's brain naturally and protectively suppresses the memories. Or denial and delusional mechanisms are so strong the addict may "refuse" to remember.

RIGIDITY AND BLAMING

David, a seminary student studying to be a priest, struggled with masturbation and homosexual attractions. His spiritual director advised him that whenever he felt sexual temptation, he should say the rosary five times, and the temptation would go away. But it didn't work. He searched for other prayers and rituals that might help, but nothing did.

David's first ministry assignment was a conservative, ethnic parish in a poor neighborhood. The men there told jokes about homosexual men, and David joined to avoid revealing his sexual orientation. One night these men began ridiculing and taunting a man who seemed to them to be gay. Then they blamed homosexuals for all the problems in the world. While David disagreed with much of what they said, he found himself getting angry and critical of the gay community. It is a common psychological dynamic to blame others for problems one experiences oneself. It is easier to be angry with others than with oneself.

David was afraid of his homosexual feelings and found it easier to go along with the crowd than to honestly face his problems. His religious rituals had failed, and he felt very lonely and isolated.

One result of sex addicts' desperate attempts to stop is that, like David, they may look for formulas to follow. They assume there is a right way and a wrong way to do things. If they could just get the formula right, then their sexual acting out would stop. This black-and-white thinking leads to rigidity. Addicts think there are good people and bad people, good groups and bad groups, and desperately want to belong to the right side. In searching for the right people and the right side, an addict may become prejudiced against others who don't belong to this group. This leads to anger against those on the "outside." "If it weren't for them, things would be right with me and the world." This is a form of self-righteousness.

Self-righteousness leads to blaming. If there is a right way of doing things, there must also be a wrong way. Other people, institutions, or events may represent the wrong way and therefore are held responsible for the bad things that happen. "It is all their fault," a sex addict might say. "If he (or she) hadn't seduced me, I wouldn't have had the affair."

Sex addicts often look to the right religious group to take away their lusts. The man who was baptized four times felt he never did find the right church. If he had, one of those baptisms would have worked, and his lust would have been removed. Some Christian addicts believe God will magically transform them into people who never experience sexual temptation. The theological correction to this misguided hope is very basic. If God did remove all of the temptations out there in the world, he would, in effect, be taking away our free will. The Bible is also consistent in teaching that temptations are opportunities to make moral choices, and when we do, we become stronger.

CODEPENDENCY

James was addicted to going to massage parlors. At first, he sought encounters with young and very attractive women. Gradually, he started seeking older prostitutes, resembling his mother. He also started to realize he wasn't so much interested in the orgasm as he was in the touching. James was looking for a mother. Every time he came out of the massage parlor, he felt frustrated and cheated, but he kept going back, always looking.

Sophia was raised in a very strict Christian home. While her father was occasionally home, he worked a lot, attended many church meetings, and had little time for Sophia. He was strict, often angry, and very critical with her. As she grew up, Sophia found herself getting attached to one man after another. She desperately needed their approval. She would do anything for them. If this included sex, so be it. Gradually, she found that she needed sex just to feel relaxed or temporarily content. Each man got bored with the relationship and left her. Every time, after intense grieving, she went out and found another. She's been married five times and has had lots of extramarital affairs.

These two cases illustrate that James and Sophia were

not only sex addicts but also codependents. They were looking for love and nurture and thought they could only find it in other people. The term codependency was originally used to refer to those who lived with and tolerated alcoholics. They were dependent on the alcoholic and therefore codependent on alcohol. Since that time, the field of codependency has come to recognize the anxiety of codependents and their desperate need for love and approval. This is the kind of need that enables them to tolerate addictive and dysfunctional behavior. It also motivates them to do anything to maintain that love and nurture. A codependent's anxiety forces them into either self-sacrificing behavior or controlling behavior. In either strategy, they try to manipulate the love and approval of someone they depend on. Codependents are deathly afraid that a person will leave them. Our research with sex addicts has found that they are too codependents at a deep emotional level.

Sex addicts crave the nurturing they have not received. They don't feel worthy of nurturance, but they seek it to fill deep holes in themselves. In looking for this connection, they become attached to people who represent this connection and become totally dependent on them. Codependency affects how sex addicts relate to all people. They sacrifice themselves, their interests, and values to please someone else.

RELATIONAL DIFFICULTIES

Sexual addiction is an intimacy disorder. Sex addicts are not able to be emotionally vulnerable with other people.

They would never tell anyone how they're honestly feeling, for they are probably not aware of how they feel themselves. Generally, their feelings are painful and to be avoided at all costs.

Sex addicts have great difficulty relating to a deep, personal level with other people. They may lie to cover up their behaviors, delude themselves and others about themselves, and generally lead a double life—one life everyone knows and the secret life only they know. These factors do not create meaningful relationships. The people sex addicts are most afraid of losing are the ones sex addicts are least likely to tell who they really are. They fear that if their loved ones really knew them, they would be rejected and abandoned.

One feature of the double life of sex addicts is their ability to tell some of their feelings to strangers yet not be able to talk at all to those close to them. This creates considerable anger for spouses, family members, and others who would like to get closer, can't, and then see their sex addicts opening up to others. But the sex addicts are less afraid of losing the stranger.

The relationships of sex addicts are often stormy and unsuccessful. They may be of a short-term nature and are certainly superficial, even though the sex addict may be very dependent on the partner. This dynamic of codependency is often called "enmeshment." A sex addict may desperately cling to someone for love, attention, and approval: "I would die if you left me."

Enmeshment can be dramatic, but it is not deeply intimate. Sex addicts may be entangled with people who need them desperately, allowing them to feel needed. Or they may be entangled with people who take care of them, thus allowing them to be irresponsible.

As part of their secret, double lives, sex addicts do not like being responsible for their time. They lie about where they've been and whom they've seen. They love free time and jobs that don't have a regular structure because it gives them the freedom to attend to their addictive activities. They also spend money on themselves and their addictive activity and don't like explaining where it went. Sex addicts may also be compulsive spenders for things other than sexual activities.

Sex addicts are "slippery." They know a lot of people, but they don't have any friends. They may be the life of the party, but no one knows them. They might have wonderful reputations, but it would shock many to know what they do sexually. They avoid accountability to anyone, so they have the freedom to pursue their addictive lifestyle.

Many sex addicts experience what is called "gender hatred," seeming to hate all men or all women. Men who sexually act out with women, for example, may be accused of hating women, particularly if the sex is exploitative, abusive, or manipulative. However, sex addicts do not actually hate all men or all women. Rather, they blame women or men for abuse suffered in childhood. If a man abused someone early in life, any man who later comes along might take on the attributes of the original abuser. The anger felt toward the original abuser is misplaced onto the current person in a process called "projection." Old feelings from previous relationships are projected onto new people and new relationships.

SEXUAL IGNORANCE AND CONFUSION

Although sex addicts have lots of sexual experiences, they may not know very much about sex. In fact, they may be full of misinformation or lack information entirely. Sex addicts typically grow up in families where sex is rarely discussed. If sex was discussed in their homes, the brief conversations almost always comprised negative messages full of the dangers of sexual immorality. The positive, healthy, and spiritual side of sex was never presented. Combine this negative teaching with the lack of positive teaching, and an undercurrent of tension develops around sexuality. Sex is "forbidden." They were left to discover what they could from their own experiences, including pornography or misguided and immoral cultural teaching.

Forbidden sex elicits curiosity and excitement, a natural and adrenaline-filled "pull" that many of us feel toward anything we know little about. In adolescence, as sexual feelings naturally develop, anyone can become frightened of sensations that are, in fact, normal. Given our cultural fascination with sexuality, this can be a very confusing time.

If sex addicts were sexually abused as children by a parent or other family member, the most significant connection with that parent or family member was sexual. If a parent is supposed to love you, and if parents are sexual with you, the conclusion is that this must be a part of the way a parent loves you. This is delusional thinking, but remember that it is a child doing it. These children may grow up to be sex addicts who think, "Sex is equal to love."

The experience of sex with a parent is frightening and painful. Sex addicts may come to believe that for sex to take place, it must be mysterious, evil, uncomfortable, and dangerous. In fact, Dr Patrick Carnes has said that for a sex addict, "For sex to be good, it has to be bad."

CROSS ADDICTIONS

As a teenager, Mike drank alcohol with his friends to loosen up before a date. When he got older, he found that drinking allowed him to be more aggressive with women. This usually got him what he wanted—sex. Even though he got married, he continued to have affairs, and his drinking progressed.

Mike's wife, who didn't know about the other women, demanded he stops drinking. Mike went to treatment for alcoholism and then regularly attended AA meetings. Although he stayed sober for years, he continued to have affairs, sometimes with other AA members. When he told his AA sponsor about his affairs, the man laughed and told Barry to do whatever it took to stop drinking.

Many sex addicts have cross addictions—they are addicted to other behaviors and substances. Sex is their primary addictive activity, but there are others. Like Mike, many sex addicts who come for treatment are already recovering alcoholics. They may have experienced many years of sobriety from alcohol. They may even have thought that if they got sober from alcohol and drugs, they would stop their sexual activities.

Tragically, however, their sexual acting out got worse when they achieved alcoholic sobriety. Some, while achieving sobriety from sex, struggle with compulsive eating. Many gain weight. Others continue to smoke heavily, spend compulsively, gamble, or watch TV incessantly. The list of possibilities is endless. I remember talking to one man who had rented sixty videos in one month, none of them R- or X-rated, from the local video store.

Sex addicts learn to escape their feelings through compulsive behavior or addictions. Many have several major addictions and a long list of minor ones. Dr Carnes has discovered in his research that the more severe the childhood abuse experience, the more likely it is that a sex addict will have multiple addictions. This makes sense. The more painful the childhood experience, the more escapes an addict needs to medicate the pain.

In recovery, sex addicts may have trouble with other addictions, and there may be significant emotional and spiritual issues left to work on. If sex is the primary way addicts escape emotional and spiritual issues, stopping sex will only bring those issues to the surface. Addicts must first learn how to deal with emotional and spiritual issues in healthy ways before dealing with the addiction itself.

Sex addicts may wonder, "When will all these addictions stop?" It is discouraging to battle many addictive behaviors, but they may suffer from what has been called an "addictive personality disorder." People who are this addictive can abuse many behaviors or substances and easily become addicted to them if they are not careful. Attention Disorders, Depression, and Anxiety Sex addicts may suffer from a wide variety of classic mental health problems. Some of these may be manifestations of the same factors that led to addiction, and some may be the result of genetic problems in the neurochemistry of the brain. This section reviews the three most common mental health conditions addicts suffer: attention disorders, depression, and anxiety.

In a recent study conducted with over 100 sex addicts, roughly 70 percent indicated Attention Deficit Disorder (ADD) might be an issue for them. ADD may represent a collection of disorders, all of them involving problems with attention, distraction, and organization.

People who have ADD may have a genetic or environmentally produced need to regulate the brain chemicals involved in the transmission and organization of thoughts. One of these chemicals, dopamine, is thought to be a primary factor in this problem. Various activities and substances, such as caffeine, nicotine, and adrenaline, can elevate dopamine. Danger and crisis stimulate adrenaline and thereby dopamine. Sexual activity and fantasy can also elevate dopamine.

This suggests that a brain that needs more dopamine is a brain that needs more stimuli. People addicted to smoking, caffeine, gambling (a dangerous or risky activity), and sex often tell me they are bored. Their brains need more stimulation. This begins to explain why many addicts have multiple addictions. They could be addicted to any substance or activity that elevates dopamine and provides the stimulation they crave. Appropriate medical treatment of attention problems can greatly impact sex addicts trying to control their sexual behaviors.

Anxiety and depression can be traced to difficult life situations but can also be traced to chemical imbalances in the brain. The consequences of sexual sin may also create anxiety and depression, but chemical imbalances can cause a person to seek relief through sexual activity.

Thus, while sexual sins can create anxiety and depression, they may also be considered the solution by addicts looking for relief.

IRRITABILITY

Sex addicts try to avoid their feelings and avoid being found out. They create enormous defenses. If anyone asks questions that come too close to the truth or simply challenges their story, addicts can become greatly irritated. Their behavior makes them angry with themselves and angry with others. Past abuse issues also create hidden resentments and anger.

Triggers that remind them of these previous events may elicit anger that appears unrelated to the significance of the event. Simple questions, insignificant events, or basic statements may incite an angry reaction that will surprise you because the reaction is out of proportion to the event.

ABUSE OF SELF OR OTHERS

If sex addicts have been abused in the past, they may do the same to others. If they have not been talked to, they won't talk to others. If they have been yelled and screamed at, they yell and scream at others. If they have been preached to, they preach to others. They abuse others in ways they were abused. Victims of this abuse may believe this is acceptable behavior, or they may be too afraid or ashamed to confront it.

Sex addicts may also abuse themselves. Their personal habits and hygiene, eating, smoking, and drinking may annoy everyone around them. They may engage in any activity or use any substance compulsively. Many sex addicts tell intimate details of their lives, except the sexual details, to strangers. Sex addicts try to get people to like them by seeming to confide in them. Sex addicts have lots of acquaintances but no friends.

RESISTANCE TO SUPERVISION OR CRITICISM

Since they hide a large part of their daily behaviors, sex addicts are not very open to criticism, whether or not it is constructively given. They may live with people who would very much like to correct their behaviors and who continue to turn up the volume of their criticisms in order to be heard. This just drives sex addicts deeper into withdrawal, for they do not want their sexual behaviors to be challenged.

USE OF SEXUAL HUMOR

Sex addicts may use sexual humor all the time. They are always teasing (which many consider sexual harassment) or telling sexual jokes. Sex addicts sexualize most situations and see some sexual humor in it. Sexual jokes can be used to recruit new sexual partners. Sex addicts can gauge the reaction of a person hearing their sexual joke, and if that reaction is favorable, the level of sexual engagement might be taken one step higher.

Sex addicts are great at double entendre—words or phrases that might have two meanings, one of them sexual. Say something in this fashion, and the sex addict will smile and point out the sexual content.

If a person says, "My friend was able to get off on time this morning," a sex addict interprets "get off" to be about orgasm and makes some sexual joke about it.

4

THE CAUSES AND PROBLEMS OF
SEXUAL ADDICTION

The mentality, thought system, and relationships that got you into addiction will keep you there unless you disentangle yourself from them.

— OCHE OTORKPA, AUTHOR: *THE NIGHT BEFORE I KILLED ADDICTION*

The first question anyone diagnosed with sexual addiction typically asks is pretty much the same: "How did I get this way?" and who could blame them? Ultimately, why a person is sexually addicted is less initially important than "how can I stop," which is the best place to begin therapy/treatment. Nevertheless, it is helpful to address the topic here, but only after noting the following: knowing why you are a sex addict will not cure or even control your sexual addiction, but it often provides meaningful shame reduction and even self-compassion.

NATURE VERSUS NURTURE

The simple truth is that some people are inherently vulnerable to addiction, and some people aren't. Consider alcohol. Nearly everyone tries alcohol at some point in their life, but only a small percentage of those folks become alcoholics. The same is true with other potentially addictive drugs and behaviors: many partake, but few become addicted.

So why can some people try it and walk away when others cannot? Surely there must be some obvious, easily spotted difference between healthy people and potential addicts? Some telltale sign that's hard to miss? Right? Wrong.

That said, there is a considerable amount of research into the causes of addiction, with scientists identifying two main categories of risk: nature and nurture.

NATURE: GENETICS AND THE RISK OF ADDICTION

Dozens of studies have identified a connection between genetic factors and susceptibility to addiction. Most of these studies focus on alcoholism, but it is not unreasonable to extend the findings to other addictions. To begin, numerous genetic mutations can either directly increase or decrease the risk of addiction, typically by altering how a specific substance (such as alcohol) is experienced and processed in the body and brain.

According to studies, naturally less reactive people (as measured by body sway) are more likely to become alcoholics. In other words, people who are genetically less susceptible to the negative side effects of alcohol can consume more longer (get higher) without falling down, getting sick, or passing out, and they are, as a result, more likely to drink alcoholically. Another study connects addiction to a specific genetic variation affecting D2 dopamine receptors, which are part of the brain's reward center. This genetic mutation, which essentially magnifies the pleasurable effects of addictive substances and behaviors, raises the risk of all addiction types, not just alcoholism.

Genetic variations can also reduce the risk of addiction. For instance, it has long been known that people of East Asian ancestry are much less likely than other groups to become alcoholics. And scientists now know why. In short, they've identified a genetic mutation (prevalent in East Asian cultures) that causes a deficiency of the aldehyde dehydrogenase enzyme, which is critical to the metabolism of alcohol. When people with this genetic mutation consume alcohol, classic hangover symptoms (headache, dehydration, nerve and tissue sensitivity, rapid heartbeat, nausea, and the like) occur almost immediately. In other words, alcohol makes these folks physically ill instead of getting them high. Alcoholism is extremely uncommon in people with this genetic make-up.

Genetic factors can also contribute to addiction indirectly. For instance, genetics are a factor in numerous psychiatric disorders: depression, anxiety, attention deficits, panic disorders, bipolar disorder, social phobia, etc. Not surprisingly, many people living with these disorders choose to self-medicate with alcohol, drugs, and intensely pleasurable behaviors. Over time this may become compulsive.

In such cases, what is genetically inherited is not a distinct response to a potentially addictive substance or behavior but rather a proclivity for addiction vulnerability. For instance, people diagnosed with bipolar disorder are much more likely than others to also have a substance use disorder. Still, this increased risk for addiction has nothing whatsoever to do with how addictive substances and behaviors are experienced in the body. Instead, it's connected to the person's desire or "need" to escape and dissociate from the shame and emotional pain of an under-lying, genetically driven psychiatric disorder.

Other examples of the indirect effect of genetics on addiction are seen when examining certain heritable personality traits such as impulsivity, risk-taking, novelty-seeking, and abnormal stress reactivity, all of which significantly increase the risk for addiction.6 In short, the genetic predisposition toward rapid, unplanned actions or reactivity without regard to potential negative consequences is closely associated with addiction. Here, it is an inherited tendency toward certain character traits that cause dangerous behaviors, one of which may be the abuse of potentially addictive substances or behaviors that leads (indirectly) to addiction. Again, the effects are not related to the physical experience of the addictive substance or behavior; rather, the effects are part of a broad spectrum of psychological and emotional predispositions that incidentally increase the risk for addiction.

NURTURE: ENVIRONMENT AND THE RISK OF ADDICTION

According to research, we cannot entirely blame addiction on genetic susceptibility; environmental factors also play a significant role. But how significant is this role, and how can we quantify it? Scientists have distinguished between nature and nurture in addiction causation studies by examining the prevalence of addiction among adopted children and twins (especially identical twins who were separated at birth and raised by different sets of parents). The relative importance of genetic risk factors versus environmental risk factors can thus be determined.

Adoption studies frequently ask, "What happens to the children of alcoholics if they are adopted into a family where neither parent drinks?" Researchers have consistently found that people with biological (not adoptive) parents who were alcoholics are much more likely to develop alcoholism. So score a point for genetics. Of course, being more likely to develop alcoholism doesn't mean that alcoholism is an absolute certainty. In fact, lots of people in these studies were not alcoholics. Plus, plenty of biological children of non-alcoholics do become alcoholics. So we can now say that environmental influences play a part.

Comparable studies have been conducted for cocaine, nicotine, and opiates with remarkably similar results, leading scientists to conclude that somewhere between 40 and 70 percent of the risk for addiction is genetic, and somewhere between 60 and 30 percent is environmental. If we wanted to use the center point of those estimates, we could say that the risk for addiction *is* 55 percent genetic and 45 percent environmental. In addition to this relatively even distribution of blame, it appears that nature can easily be usurped by nurture (again potentially epigenetics).

For instance, abused or neglected children have an incredibly high risk for addiction (and other adult-life psychological issues) regardless of genetic influences. Furthermore, the more times a child is traumatized, the greater the likelihood of adverse reactions, such as addiction, later in life.

Early exposure to an addictive drug or activity is another reasonably common environmental risk factor. Numerous studies have found that the lower the age of first use, the higher the likelihood of addiction. This is true with all forms of addiction, including sexual addiction. Whether sex was vilified or glorified, many sex addicts were exposed to it at an unusually early age. One recent survey of adult sex addicts found that 41 percent were using pornography before the age of twelve. Keep in mind that Internet porn was not nearly as available when today's adult sex addicts were twelve or younger, so kids had to dig hard for it, or, more likely, they had to be subjected to it unintentionally or intentionally—a potentially traumatic experience in any case.

Sometimes the age of first use (drugs or behaviors) and familial instability (including a family history of mental illness and addiction) are directly related, as addictive substances or activities are readily available within the home. Other environmental risk factors (such as inconsistent parenting, neglect, abuse, etc.) may play a larger role in the development of addiction in such cases.

SEXUAL ABUSE, SEXUAL SHAME, AND SEXUAL ADDICTION

Undoubtedly, childhood sexual abuse, whether a single incident or chronic, leaves its victims with feelings of confusion and shame. This is true whether the abuse is overt, meaning "hands-on," or covert, as occurs when a parent "emotionally partners" with a child. Exacerbating matters is the fact that childhood sexual abuse is often coupled with other forms of early-life trauma, such as emotional, psychological, or physical neglect and abuse, creating layers of traumatic experience and various forms of shame—though sexual shame is nearly always the most powerful.

Frequently, sexually shamed children begin to self-medicate their emotional discomfort relatively early in life, usually during adolescence but sometimes even before. After all, body image issues, shame about being looked at or touched inappropriately, and feeling "icky" about too much trust and affection can all begin *very early* in childhood. It is typical to see these emotionally challenged children seeking solace (by early adolescence) via drug and alcohol abuse. That said, many children also learn (or are taught) that they can self-soothe with sexual behaviors (including sexual fantasy and masturbation), usually by eroticizing and reenacting some aspect of their sexual trauma. In fact, self-soothing through the eroticized reenactment of trauma is relatively common.

Unfortunately, while these self-soothing sexual activities can be distracting at the moment, they appear to intensify preexisting shame and emotional distress, leading to an increased desire for escape and dissociation. As such, many deeply sexually shamed "sexual trauma survivors" find themselves mired in an addictive cycle of self-hatred and sexual shame, ameliorated by sexual fantasy and activity, followed by still more self-hatred and sexual shame. In other words, their escapist addictive sexual fantasies and habits inherently and automatically create a desire for more of the same. As you may recall from Chapter 1, this is the foundation of the sex-addiction cycle.

UNDERSTANDING COVERT INCEST

Covert incest, also referred to as emotional incest, is when a parent, stepparent, or other long-term caregiver uses or abuses a child in an indirect, sexualized, or romanticized way. In contrast to overt sexual abuse, which involves hands-on sexual contact, covert abuse involves less direct forms of sexuality— Sexuality that is implied or suggested emotionally rather than overtly acted out. A child is thus used for parental emotional fulfillment, being forced to support the adult by acting as a trusted confidante or an "emotional spouse." Though there may be little to no direct sexual activity, these overly entwined relationships have a sexualized undertone, with the parent expressing excessive graphic-verbal interest in the child's physical development and sexual characteristics or betraying the child's boundaries through sexualized conversations, exhibitionism, voyeurism, and inappropriate sharing of intimate stories or images.

Covert incest often occurs when parents have distanced themselves from one another both physically and emotionally. One or the other parent begins to place their adult emotional needs on their child, using the child as a kind of surrogate partner. Some parents may tie their own self-esteem to the child's academic, sports or other success. Either way, the child's developmental needs tend to be ignored, and emotional growth (especially in the area of healthy sexual and romantic attachment) can be profoundly stunted. Often, the perpetrating adult is usually completely unaware of the emotional damage he or she creates by using their child as an emotional object, rather than turning to other adults for support.

And typically, for many trauma survivors without concrete, identifiable trauma stories (involving: hitting, rape, profound neglect, violence, etc.), this kind of emotional damage can be hard to identify. Clients in treatment will say things like, "Once Dad left, I got all of Mom's attention; she was with me constantly and told me everything."

They often feel like they got a pretty good deal, but in reality, being responsible for a parent's emotional needs at such a young age can be very damaging to a child and bodes poorly for their future relationships and sexuality.

Most covert incest survivors initially resist the notion that they have been sexually abused because they were never actually touched sexually by the perpetrator. However, these relationships are indeed sexualized. Essentially, a child in these circumstances is sexualized and treated as an adult partner. Therefore he or she is deprived of healthy attachment bonds, stable emotional growth, and many other basics of childhood development. In place of healthy development, the child is taught that his or her value is based not on who he or she is as a person but on how much they can please, amuse, and bond with the care-taker. As a result, covert incest survivors typically respond in the same ways as survivors of overt (hands-on) sexual abuse, with many of the following adult-life symptoms and consequences:

- Characterlogical and personality (ego) problems
- Addiction and compulsivity
- Difficulty developing and maintaining long-term intimacy
- Narcissism and angry emotional reactivity
- Shame and feelings of inadequacy
- Dissociation
- Difficulties with self-care (emotional or physical)
- Love/hate relationships, especially with spouses and family
- Inappropriate bonding or overly distancing with their child (intergenerational abuse)
- Adult intimacy disorders

Covert incest is so pervasive and damaging that it frequently goes unnoticed, even in treatment therapy settings. Only when we delve beneath the surface do we discover the links between covertly incestuous behaviors and adult intimacy and addiction issues, including sexual addiction.

SEXUAL ADDICTION: THE PERFECT STORM

Sex addicts, like all other addicts, are subject to a combination of genetic and environmental risk factors. For instance, a combination of genetic predisposition, abusive, alcoholic, or mentally ill parents, childhood trauma, and early exposure occur relatively often, creating a witch's brew of ongoing life problems: not just addiction, but numerous other social, emotional, and psychological issues. Given this, it is clear that any discussion about the possible causes of sexual addiction is not so much an argument of nature versus nurture as an examination of how the two factors come together to influence individual behavior and response. In short, addictive disorders of all types, sexual addiction included, are driven by genetics and environmental factors. When early-life sexual trauma (overt or covert) is part of the mix, the odds of sexual addiction versus another addiction greatly increase.

❦ 5 ❦

LEVELS OF SEXUAL ADDICTION

We live in an era when the "joy of sex" is seen as everyone's deserving pursuit. To be celibate is almost to be suspect. As part of the sexual revolution, inhibitions and hang-ups are discarded. In many ways, this shift in our cultural mores constitutes a breakthrough in exploring human sexuality. It is an essential antidote to the proscriptive past and a significant acknowledgment of our sexual nature. As in all major culture changes, there are excesses. Our preoccupation with sex pervades almost all facets of our contemporary lifestyles.

In an age when the variety and quality of sexual experience are highly valued, there is a group that is often overlooked: those who are sexually compulsive in ways they do not want to be. To think of sexual addicts as simply guilt-ridden because of their sexual behavior is to misunderstand the nature of the addiction.

This point of view assumes that addicts need to be freer and enjoy their sexuality and that they feel bad as a result of unhelpful scruples and misinformation. Masturbation, for example, is now widely accepted as a developmental stage and a natural expression of personal sexuality. Accepting his desire to masturbate is no longer enough for the man who masturbates so frequently that he has occasionally severely injured his penis. His masturbation is seriously affecting his life and causing harm to his body.

Sexual addicts are aware of the pain and consequences. They are aware of their own emptiness. If they're lucky, they'll be aware of the exploitation and harm they're causing others. They are always afraid of being exposed because of their obsessive behavior. This is not to suggest that sexual addicts are uninhibited and free of hang-ups.

On the contrary, they often do come from highly proscriptive families and carry damaging myths inside them. Part of recovery always is restructuring the belief system by acquiring adequate information and accepting one's own sexuality. However, the first task of recovery is to focus on the uncontrollable behavior.

When discussing sexual addiction, it is necessary to recognize that not everyone who has a regrettable sexual experience is an addict. There are people who have regrets over specific events, realizing that their sexual behavior on a given occasion was not in their best interest. They add it to their experience and simply do not repeat it.

There are numbers who have abused their sexuality. Going on a sexual binge, for example, might occur after graduation or in retaliation to a lover's indiscretion.

There are also those who have episodes of compulsivity. Those who study middle-age transition, the famous "middlescence," note the sexual bingeing which can occur at that time. Also, it is often seen as a post-divorce pattern. The divorced person, who is suddenly free from marital obligations, may experiment to excess.

Adolescents struggle with the ferocity of their developing sexuality. Adolescent sexual expression is a major contention factor between peer support and parental prohibition. Identity formation includes experimentation and exploration. Internalizing appropriate rules and boundaries requires learning from youthful enthusiasm. In that sense, adolescence is similar to the "middle adolescent" search for self. As a result, episodes of sexual excess may only indicate a shift in one's life circumstances.

Also, there are those who may have a problem, but not necessarily an addiction. Let's consider an example, say, a college professor nationally recognized for his careful scholarship. On occasion, he had the urge to go to a porno theater. While watching the movie, he would masturbate, which he found very exciting. When leaving, however, an immense depression would always come over him. He felt degraded. He worried about being recognized or, worse, arrested.

He would always vow not to repeat the experience. Over a period of eight years, he had done it four to five times. The professor's problem has some important parallels with sexual addiction. The excitement/depression scenario is a common story for the addict. So are breaking the rules and the excitement of the illicit.

Also, the vow to quit or make it the last time is part and parcel of the addiction. Yet, he is not an addict. This is not to minimize his problem, which is painful and abusive. He runs the risk of adverse consequences, but, in general, his life has not become unmanageable. In short, he has not entered the addict's world. If the professor had experienced periods in which he repeated the behavior frequently with damaging results, he would clearly have an addictive pattern.

Many addicts describe their experiences as episodic, meaning they have periodic binges that have serious consequences for their work, relationships, and self-esteem.

They may have extended periods of no problems in between binges. Being able to stop for a short period of time gives the addict the illusion of control, making it more difficult for the addict to recognize that there is a problem. However, over time, a pattern of bingeing reveals an unmistakable addiction. For some addicts, bingeing becomes so frequent that it becomes a habit.

If the professor's situation were changed again and his visits to the theater were a part of a much larger picture, including massage parlors, strip shows, and multiple affairs, his actions also would have a very different meaning. A clear case of addiction can emerge when other forms of sexual compulsiveness are considered as well. The assessment of the addiction's extent or intensity is complete only with first examining the varieties of sexual addiction.

LEVELS OF ADDICTION

Addicts often comment in group therapy that they are astounded at how similar their experiences were, even though what they did was vastly different. While the varieties of addiction are great, the sexual addiction cycle described in chapter one is common.

Categorizing the various forms of sexual compulsiveness into different groups helps in several ways.

First, grouping provides a perspective of the wide range of sexual behaviors in which addiction can thrive. From this perspective, addicts can make a better inventory of the scope of their addiction.

Second, some sexual behavior involves great danger, breaks the law, or victimizes others. For the addicts, these behaviors show greater powerlessness and unmanageability. Risking greater consequences for a more exciting high indicates an escalation of the addiction.

Finally, every addict must understand his or her own unique pattern of sexually compulsive behavior. Subtle differences are extremely important for addicts, especially in early recovery. For example, strategies for avoiding unique cues and rituals which initiate the addictive cycle can be developed once a pattern is identified.

To interrupt the addictive cycle, the addict must understand his or her pattern of behavior. Creating a framework for the behavior has made that task easier. A workable structure that helps identify patterns is viewing the addiction as operating at three levels.

The first level, Level One, contains behaviors that are regarded as normal, acceptable, or tolerable. Examples include masturbation, homosexuality, and prostitution.

Level Two, by contrast, extends to those behaviors which are clearly victimizing and for which legal sanctions are enforced. These are generally seen as nuisance offenses such as exhibitionism or voyeurism.

Level Three behaviors, such as incest, child molestation, or rape, have grave consequences for victims and legal consequences for addicts. At this level, compulsivity represents a severe progression of the addiction.

Suggesting three levels does not mean that addicts cannot destroy their lives with Level One behavior. Many addicts have done just that without ever venturing into Levels Two or Three. It would be unusual, however, for an addict to be compulsive at Levels Two or

Three without a significant amount of compulsivity at Level One. Most rare is the addict who simply focuses on only one form of sexual compulsiveness. But that, too, does happen. Within a level or across levels, the addict must understand the full range of possibilities.

LEVEL ONE

Level One behaviors have in common general cultural acceptance. If some are regarded as inappropriate or even illegal, the reality is that widespread practice conveys public tolerance. The other common characteristic is that each can be devastating when done compulsively. Even the healthiest forms of human sexual expression can devolve into self-defeating behaviors or, in the worst-case scenario, victimization of others.

Masturbation

Masturbation is an essential part of being a sexual person. Nurturing oneself, exploring sexual needs and fantasies, and establishing basic self-knowledge are vital contributions that masturbation makes to sexual identity. As sexual therapists are keenly aware, it is more difficult to have a vital sexual relationship without these factors. In fact, for people who suffer from sexual dysfunction, therapy often involves a careful rebuilding of a patient's attitudes and beliefs around masturbation.

For the addict, however, masturbation becomes a degrading event. Masturbating 4 to 5 times every day for years on end becomes a secret life. It is the central part of every day. At the least feeling of frustration or loneliness, the addict struggles to find a private place to masturbate. Unlocking the office door, walking out of the bathroom, or driving in the car, the addict is certain that no one else is as obsessed as he is.

Part of that certainty comes from the collection of judgments and beliefs he holds to be true about masturbation. Messages from parents, family, and church have left no doubt that it is a character flaw. As a result, the addict may carry some equation in his or her head: masturbation equals failure. Masturbation equals a loss of manhood. Masturbation is not feminine. Masturbation equals punishment.

One addict tells a story about his Catholic upbringing. Each Saturday, his father would ask if the boy had to go to confession. Since masturbation was a sin, both boy and father knew what had to be confessed. The father would talk to the boy about how he would become a man when he conquered his urges. The boy would sit in his shame. He dreaded Saturdays.

It later turned out that the father was simply telling his own belief his own myth to the boy. The father was a compulsive masturbator who believed that his problem was simply a lack of self-control.

In his desperation to prevent the same pain for his son, the father relayed the myth which locked him into his own addiction. (The same image of ideal manliness, which added to the father's shame, was passed on to his son.) Paradoxically, he recreated the same addictive system for his son out of love. As addicts go, this is a common story.

The son translated the message in a particularly damaging way. He felt that God would punish him for his masturbation. In fact, he believed that nothing would go right for him for the twenty-four hours following each time he masturbated. Given the power of his expectations and his daily masturbation, his life was an unending cycle of failure and disappointments. His compulsive masturbating was central to the self-fulfilling prophecy of God's punishment.

Heterosexual Relationships

Addiction can take a variety of forms in a heterosexual relationship. Addiction is present at the most basic level when one partner sacrifices important aspects of the relationship in the service of sexual needs. When a spouse or significant other begins to feel victimized by the other's sexuality, this is a red flag. (When exploited feelings are dismissed, the warning becomes stronger.)

Relationship needs are traded for sexual needs when the spouse's feelings are ignored. There are times in every relationship when sexual needs aren't met. The addict, on the other hand, turns the other person into an obsession. The relationship is conditional on sexual performance for the partner. Both partners miss out on the fun, intimacy, and freedom of mutual loving sexual play. Sexuality loses its ability to nurture, grow, and improve one's quality of life. Addiction weakens, demoralizes, and depletes a relationship.

Some addicts seek solace in a number of different relationships. Consider a woman whose loneliness is exacerbated by a seemingly endless string of one-night stands. She can't seem to stop the blur of faces and bodies, no matter how hard she tries. Take, for example, the man who rarely has just one relationship but is "meaningfully" involved in several at the same time. He may admit to not even liking his sexual partners if he stops, to be honest. It was a delusion to believe that the relationships were meaningful in order to get into bed.

The question isn't whether or not it's possible to love more than one person at the same time. The issue here is the fear of having to live without sex.

For the desperate addict, cruising is one of the ultimate activities. The contrast of excitement and loneliness characterizes hustling in bars, streets, and parties. Will I be chosen? Will I be successful? Even the prospect is exhilarating. The sadness is masked by memories of successful forays, the smells, the music, and the adventures. Professional, business, and educational settings are places where people seek sexual gratification. The void that sex tries to fill, however, remains the same.

For example, Chris, an addict whose cruising was intertwined with her work as an urban planning consultant. Her ability to clearly articulate the complex problems in her field, combined with her charisma and attractiveness, made her a sought-after speaker. Seminars, conferences, and workshops were a regular part of her schedule. They were just a front for her real life. Her sexual opportunities grew as a result of her travels. In each of the cities she visited on a regular basis, she had ongoing relationships. Even more common were one-night stands. In retrospect, she would later say that traveling was sexual. It began the moment she stepped onto the plane. Her profession acted as a powerful catalyst for her addiction.

Cruising as a source of sexual gratification can even occur within the context of marriage, with tragic consequences. Their friends thought Fred and Liza were the perfect couples. Their addiction problems began when they were both in graduate school. They were sweethearts at fourteen and married at twenty. Liza had confessed to Fred that she had been picked up and "made" one night after being at a bar. Fred's response was unexpected. He was enthralled by it and made ardent love to her. He asked her to repeat the process with the same results. Soon their lovemaking became frequent that Liza would seduce a man, tell Fred all about it, and then make love with Fred.

As the excitement wore off, Fred urged Liza to bring the men home. As he and his wife watched the men, Fred would masturbate. He eventually became more involved in orchestrating the activities that became increasingly degrading to Liza.

After a few years, their married life became centered on these events. When they finally sought help, the part of their story that stood out was how much they both wanted to stop. They had even made joint efforts to stop, particularly when Liza was hurt. The central part of their recovery was in reclaiming their very real love of one another.

Prostitution

Every now and then, a vice squad will close in on an outcall service that has made prostitutes available to customers by phone. Records are seized. A chill goes through the city. Eight to ten thousand men wonder if their names were kept on file. The paper accentuates this fear by printing the police comment that the list of patrons included prominent government officials, religious leaders, and businessmen. Each patron, in his shame, fears that his name has surfaced. All rehearse confessions and stories for their bosses and wives. The public feels sensation and fear, glimpsing for a moment the large network of people who make prostitution a part of their lives.

Prostitution appears in many forms. Some outcall services are so large they have representatives in the major metropolitan areas of the country. Simply call a toll-free number. Massage, rap, and sauna parlors will charge their services on major credit cards.

Many metropolitan hotels are routinely worked by young, often beautiful women. Businesses hire public relations "consultants." Listening to a CB radio, one quickly becomes aware of vans and pickups driven by women with handles like "Bunny" or "Snuggles." They work the nation's truck stops and rest areas. These forms of the "oldest profession" do not generate a public reaction.

Somehow, concern is generated only for the streetwalker who works the bars and streets under the tyranny of a pimp. Or the adolescent runaway who ends up a prostitute to survive. Or the young boy who works as a "chicken" in gay cruising areas. The issue of whether prostitution is a victimless crime goes beyond the scope of this section. Our focus of concern is on the addict whose involvement with prostitution is crippling his or her life.

Addicts who use the Twelve Steps will often joke about going to "Johns Anonymous" because of the prevalence of prostitution in the sexual addiction and the usage by prostitutes of the word "John" to describe their customers. Addicts like prostitutes because it is an immediate fix with few entanglements. Often it is anonymous. Yet, the consequences of prostitution are high. The lies often are elaborate. There is risk of disease. There is the possibility of it becoming public knowledge. Yet, the biggest factor for most addicts is the expense. A habit of three to four visits a week is expensive to sustain. One addict, a physician, used up all the equity from the sale of an expensive home in prostitution.

Even more, for family men, lies are required to explain where the money has gone. When addicts tell about themselves, their stories are frequently punctuated with deep sobs as they tell of the times when they would come home after spending a hundred dollars on a prostitute, only to realize that their children and wives were doing without something they needed. However, as in all addictions, painful realization does not stop compulsive behavior.

Our understanding of prostitutes needs to be expanded. We are aware of women who sell their services because of financial desperation or a drug habit. We also know the impact of sexual and physical abuse from which prostitutes recycle the dramas of their own early family experiences. We know about runaways and pimps. We have even heard of happy hookers. Less aware are we of the woman addict who buries her pain with sexual obsession.

Prostitution, even part-time, can be a way to get paid for a compulsive sexual need. Some prostitutes who fail to understand this part of themselves are very difficult to stop.

Homosexuality

Recent decades have witnessed the struggle of homosexual people to establish themselves in the eyes of the straight community. Despite increased acceptance, there remains in our culture shame and judgment of what is seen as "perverse." Our lack of knowledge is underlined by increasing efforts to understand the origins of homosexuality.

For gay or lesbian persons who are also sexual addicts, compulsivity simply compounds problems of acceptance and shame. For the sexual addict whose self-image is already marginal, adding the problems of sexual identity intensifies all sexual issues.

The gay man who has eight to ten sexual encounters with different partners during a week's time has little chance to develop a real sense of self because of his loneliness and isolation. If those encounters are under degrading or even dangerous circumstances, self-image suffers further.

For example, Jim, a Lutheran seminarian, went to school full-time and worked part-time as a parish youth director. He was sensitive, intelligent, and committed to his career. He was also driven by his sexual compulsion. His pattern was to frequent at night a well-known park area by a local river which was known as a gay "cruising" area. He would stand by the same tree each time and allow himself to be picked up. His sexual contacts were in the dark with strangers. He always felt humiliated. One time he was severely beaten.

What prompted Jim to seek help was not a "river" incident. Rather, he was sexual with one of the young adults in the parish he served who had visited him at his apartment. He became aware of how vulnerable he was and, in his fear, sought therapy. Once in therapy, he realized he really had two issues. First, his homosexual orientation would be a problem in his ministry. And second, his sexual compulsiveness was an obstacle to developing significant relationships. His issues around homosexuality were compounded by his sexual addiction.

The addiction is even more complicated for men who consider themselves heterosexual but are compulsive only in homosexual ways. For example, during a particularly stressful period, Steve, a happily married man, got involved with a man in a restroom in his office building. He had the same experience a few days later. Within a few months, he was a regular in his neighborhood's "hot johns." He eventually expanded into porno shops, where he met men in movie booths. This lasted a total of four years.

Two events brought Steve to therapy. The first was that he met his brother walking through the booths at the porno store. He immediately acknowledged to himself that his brother was as troubled as he. Second, while traveling, he had sex with a man in a service station toilet while his wife and kids waited in the car. During therapy, Steve realized that seeing his brother recalled all those heavily weighted family messages he carried about sexuality and homosexuality. Finally, he had to recognize that his family life was not happy. Comfortable, but not intimate. The service station episode simply underscored that he was lonely in the midst of those he loved.

The Level One Addict

Level One addicts seldom stay with one behavior category. More common would be an addict for whom prostitution, affairs, visits to porno shops, and occasional visits to hot johns form an overall picture of obsession. The accumulated effect is that the addiction can become the center of the addict's life, rooted in a complex malaise of deceit, isolation, and shame.

Because their behavior is not constant, many Level One addicts believe they can control it. They have episodes in which they simply binge sexually. They then come to a halt for weeks or even months. A salesman, for example, may only use prostitutes when he travels. In town, he perceives his life as "normal." Vows to quit made upon return from his last trip are forgotten with the next. Because of the appearance of "normalcy," he rationalizes that he can handle his behavior and that it has no impact on his life.

Yet, he truly has a secret world where damaging consequences subtly overtake him. Normal persons do not carry the secrets and shame he does. He does not stop because he cannot. The problem for the Level One addicts is that they can rationalize that they are not much different from most folks. While they feel unique in desperateness and obsession, the sexual behavior creates few real social consequences. Yet, the addicts pay a personal toll in increasing pain and loneliness. However, the next level of addiction involves clear violations of cultural norms and, therefore, greater risk. Also, greater excitement.

LEVEL TWO

Level two addictive behaviors are intrusive enough to warrant harsh legal penalties. When actively prosecuted, exhibitionism, voyeurism, indecent phone calls, and indecent liberties are all punished. However, both prosecutors and the general public regard these acts as nuisance offenses. The offenders are seen as pathetic and usually unable to establish effective relationships.

Yet, there are victims, and there are sanctions. The consequences and danger are clearly part of the addictive process. The victimization of someone is a feature shared by all Level Two obsessions.

Exhibitionism

According to Gene Abel of the New York State Psychiatric Institute, exhibitionist clients have been exposed two to three hundred times with few or no arrests. There is consensus about the reasons. Fear of reporting, indifference, and cynicism about impact are a few. One of the main factors is that victims seldom obtain detailed descriptions. The result is that an addict's actions can go unchecked for quite some time. Therefore, what starts as some experimentation can quickly become a flourishing addiction with little interference.

Stereotypically, a flasher is a person who wears a raincoat on sunny days. However, the truth is that exhibitionists are remarkably diverse in their methods, such as:

- Driving or parking in a car with pants pulled down.
- Leaving the pants' zipper open and standing in an elevator, on a street, or in a phone booth.
- Having a "strategic" hole in a pair of jeans or shorts.
- Wearing swimming trunks without liners.
- Leaving curtains "inadvertently" ajar in bedroom or bathroom.
- Ringing a doorbell in a secluded doorway and exposing when it is answered.
- Walking exposed in shopping malls, campuses, open areas.
- Approaching a building with large windows such as a library or an apartment building and exposing through the window.

Actually, there are many people who witness an act of exposure who are either unaware of the exhibitionist's intention or dismiss their own judgment as "paranoia." To expose without raising alarm becomes part of the challenge for the exhibitionist. It also limits the consequences of the addiction.

The method involving the highest risk for the exposer is the use of an automobile. Victims often have sufficient presence of mind to get a license number. Yet, driving is a very common practice. The addict can escape quickly in a car if necessary and cover more ground searching for women. Exhibitionists who drive while exposing almost invariably report car accidents as one of the consequences of their addiction. They are totally entranced by their approach to their victim and simply do not watch where they are going.

For the exhibitionist whose pattern involves driving, simply entering a car becomes a cue to start the ritual. Scanning streets for potential "scores" becomes almost part of driving. Certain streets and areas become routes that are regularly checked. The addict cannot trust that he will arrive at his intended destination because driving itself has become a real part of the ritual. Some addicts count making it to work on time a major victory, for once an addict begins cruising, three to six hours may go by before he stops.

The human cost is incredible. Exhibitionists lead double lives. They are constantly terrified that someone who has seen them in their street roles will recognize them in their "other" lives. Worse, they judge themselves by the same standards society uses as weird, nuisance perverts. That judgment is not accurate since there is trauma for the victim. Being accosted by an exposer can be very damaging and frightening. Even most exhibitionists carry an image of a person's face whom they know they have hurt. Both society and the addict underestimate the danger and the cost of the addiction.

Voyeurism

"Peeping Toms," like flashers, have their stereotypes. The ineffectual bachelor peering into the neighboring apartment via the telescope may seem harmless. For voyeur addicts, however, peeping is usually not their only compulsive behavior. They often become involved in other addictive behaviors such as pornography, movies, and strip shows. Moreover, being quite inventive in voyeurism is characteristic. Addicts have many stories about heat vents, mirrors, and cameras. Some of their efforts involve great risk, including peering into house or apartment windows or even hiding in closets.

Over and above the obvious costs, including the risk of arrest, most voyeurs agree one of the biggest losses is time. Watching a window for three or four hours, often under very awkward circumstances in the hope of glimpsing ninety seconds of nudity, is insane to even to the addict. Voyeurs report that while waiting, they often struggle with themselves asking, "Why am I doing this?"

They make a commitment to stop waiting by a certain time if nothing happens. Yet, the time comes and goes. They sit and continue to wait until either something happens or obviously nothing will. Each episode is followed by depression and pain. The loss of time and energy, the deep embarrassment about being a voyeur, the self-hatred at being unable to control oneself combine to keep an addict absolutely isolated. There is one simple way to alleviate the pain temporarily. Do it again.

As with most addicts, the voyeur is sustained by excitement. He waits in a trance-like state, with energies focused on the waiting. Totally absorbed, the addict loses all contact with reality, save for focus of the addiction. Cares, worries, deadlines, and responsibilities are suspended for a blessed moment. The mood-altering qualities of the experience are enhanced by the intrusive, the stolen, the illicit parts of the behavior. Objectively, the voyeur could go to the local topless bar and see more with less risk and discomfort. He could have sex with someone who wants to have sex with him. Or he could also pay for sex. However, it is not the same.

The thrill of illicit victimization stems from the addicts' rage. Breaking the rules is a form of retaliation for both real and imagined wrongs. The addicts' anger is fueled by a set of beliefs, family messages, and self-judgments that they use to interpret the world. The majority of addicts do not associate their behavior with anger. The trance's excitement and arousal and the rest of the pain block the feelings.

The more rage and pain there is, the more excitement is needed to block it. This dynamic is critical to comprehending how escalation occurs in the addictive process. If the current behavior within the addictive cycle no longer provides the excitement required to block the pain, something riskier is attempted. A good example is an addict who is a combination voyeur-exhibitionist.

The Voyeur-Exhibitionist

Voyeurism and exhibitionism often go together. The connecting link is masturbation. For the voyeur, masturbating while watching is another way of enhancing the excitement. The addict finds a position in which he can watch attractive women walk by but in which he cannot be seen. This is usually a car, a first-floor restroom, office, or bedroom, or even a portable outhouse of the type found in beaches, parks, and rest areas. The thrill is in ejaculating within a few feet of a woman without her knowledge. Masturbating in front of her is but a fragile step away.

Indecent Calls and Liberties

When an addict calls a woman, he or she makes suggestive statements, asks intrusive or embarrassing sexual questions, or verbally assaults her. Compared with the voyeur-exhibitionist, the difference is that victimization occurs visually with one and orally with the other. Masturbation serves as an important link here as well. Addicts will start by masturbating while talking on the phone to a woman who is not aware of it. However, attempts to be more explicit about the sexual intrusion soon follow.

Indecent liberties are inappropriate touches sometimes referred to as mini rapes. Here, too, addicts follow a path of escalating addiction. In the press of a crowded subway or shopping mall, the brush of a hand against a thigh or breast can be regarded as accidental. In the rush, it is hard not to bump into someone.

Addicts tell stories about what they would do to "have accidents" in the company of their spouses or children. Loved ones become a cover, the incongruity of which adds to the addicts' shame. All the ingredients are present: the stolen, the illicit, the exciting.

Escalation with indecent liberties takes a significant departure. Touching others with their knowledge but without their permission is the next step.

LEVEL THREE

Some of our most important boundaries are violated, which is a common feature of Level Three behavior. Rape, incest, and child molesting are basic transgressions of laws designed to protect the vulnerable. There is little compassion or understanding for someone compulsive at this level. Yet, addiction exists here too. Whether or not there should be compassion or understanding is another issue. That addiction exists here is a fact.

Molesting and Incest

The addict who focuses on children usually has suffered some interruption in their own development while growing up. There is a part of the addict which is not any older than the victim.

Actual behavior may span all three levels of addiction, including compulsive masturbation with child pornography, child prostitution, voyeuristic and exposing behavior with children, as well as molestation. There are child molesters who are compulsive with adults as well. In those situations, the addict prefers either child before adult or adult before child. Further complicating factors reside in the sexual identity of the addict, i.e., man or woman, homosexual or heterosexual.

Child sexual abuse has a long history that goes far beyond the scope of this book. As our awareness grows of its extent, the more we know of its damage. Abuse is a major factor in the transmission of sexual compulsivity from one generation to the next. This is especially true in families where incest is present.

What a child learns from a parent is how to have a relationship. When a parent is sexual with a child, the child concludes at a fundamental level that in order to have a relationship, one has to be sexual. Thus, all relationships become sexualized. Fathers and mothers are naturally attracted to their children. One of the gifts of parenthood is not to act on those feelings. Those who argue for the right of children to be sexual with their parents miss the developmental point.

Vern was intensely active sexually with his two daughters for an eight-year period. The fact did not come out until his family was brought in during his alcoholism treatment. He knew his behavior was wrong and had struggled repeatedly to stop. As part of his therapy, Vern had to confront the fact that he had been sexually abused by both his mother and father. When talking with his dad, who was still alive, he discovered that the abuse transcended four generations. His father, too, had been abused. Vern also acknowledged that his sexual addiction extended to pornography, many affairs, and extensive involvement with prostitutes.

A situation similar to incest exists for professionals such as physicians or therapists whose patients are like children in their vulnerability. For the professional to be sexual with them also is to betray trust. In reality, the sexual addict who exploits professional-client relationships is committing a type of incest. Remember, however, behavior by itself does not make an addict.

Further, to have feelings of attraction for a child (or a client) does not constitute addiction. Even to act on those feelings, as damaging as that would be, does not make an addict. Addicts are people who cannot stop their behavior which is crippling them and those around them.

COROLLARIES OF THE LEVELS OF ADDICTION

The levels of addiction are arbitrary concepts. They serve, however, to show the wide range of behavior included in sexual addiction. While our discussion did not extend to every possible form of the addiction (e.g., bestiality, sadomasochism, and fetishism were omitted), the levels provide a basic strategy for understanding any sexually compulsive behavior. Most importantly, the levels make explicit the pattern created by the relationship between behaviors.

6

THE ADDICT'S BELIEF SYSTEM:
HOW AN ADDICT THINKS AND
BEHAVES

L et us use men as an example. If a man comes from a family in which he feels bad about himself, has little confidence, women would want to be with him, and he would believe that sex is the one comfort he cannot do without. Place that same man in a culture that makes women into sexual objects, and addiction will thrive.

The belief system, the impaired thinking, preoccupation and obsession, and ritualization are all enhanced by cultural perceptions. People overlook powerlessness because it is the nature of men "to be carried away." As long as we de-personalize sex, men do not have to be responsible.

Addicts often talk about the difficulty of recovery. They live in a culture in which a major part of advertising efforts portrays sex as central to good life. Addicts already struggle with personal obsession. They have to struggle with cultural, sexual obsession as well. If the male addict went to men friends to share how he wanted to stop having affairs or seeing prostitutes, his friends might well respond, "Why would you want to do that?"

Part of the male image is the conquest of women. Another part of the image, which advertising people know, is that men are susceptible to sexual overtures. They are perceived as powerless when it comes to their sexual needs. They will do what they can "to get it," and the best man is the one who succeeds in doing just that.

These perceptions result from the fusion of faulty core beliefs with dysfunctional cultural attitudes. The perceptions reflect the addicts' low self-worth and alienation and their basic confusion that sexual expression will relieve their personal pain. Also reflected are the conflicting cultural roles of men and women.

Stated in its most extreme form of dysfunction: women decide whether men will have sex or not. Men control economic security. For the addict, two themes emerge. The first is an overwhelming need for sexual contact. He experiences this need in an environment that bombards him with sexual titillation from newsstands, television, and sales campaigns that use sex to market products. The second is a profound hopelessness that other people will not meet his sexual needs. Or if they are partially met, it will not be enough. Seduction, illicit behavior, and manipulation all become options and also add excitement to the addictive cycle. For some addicts, the ultimate bind emerges when you believe you must have it, but no one will give it to you. That profound sense of powerlessness can escalate to the use of force and the victimization of others.

The levels of addiction described in the previous

chapter provide a framework for understanding how the sexual addict's victimization of others is connected to his powerlessness. The more he believes he cannot influence his relationships with women, the more likely he is to perform Level Two and Three behaviors. Built on the premise that he is powerless, the addict's belief system becomes an elaborate structure of myths and delusions which he sees as reality, but in fact:

- Diminish his self-worth.
- Limit his possibilities in relationships.
- Use his needs to justify his victimization.
- Connect sexuality with survival.

The more dysfunctional the belief system, the higher the probability the addict's pattern of sexual compulsiveness will include the types of victimization found in Levels Two and Three. All addicts must alter their fundamental "core beliefs" in order to recover. In that sense, they are no different from anyone else who is dealing with personal issues.

THE MALE SEXUAL ADDICT'S BELIEFS ABOUT SEX, MEN, AND WOMEN

THE CORE BELIEFS	THE ADDICT'S SELF-PERCEPTION
1. Self-image: I'm completely an unworthy and bad person.	I am not attractive, personally or physically. A woman would not choose me.
2. Relationships: Nobody is going to love me the way I am.	I will have to convince a woman to be with me.
3. Needs: My needs will never be met if I have to rely on others.	My needs can only be met by luck or chance, careful strategizing, or the accumulation of money or power.
4. Sexuality: My primary need is sex.	I need sex all the time, cannot get enough, and must not pass up any opportunities. I am the only one who needs sex this much.

THE CORE BELIEFS	THE ADDICT'S PERCEPTION OF MEN	THE ADDICT'S PERCEPTION OF WOMEN
1. Self-image: I'm completely an unworthy and bad person.	Other men are more attractive, more successful, and more likely to be chosen by women.	Women choose men who are not like me. They prefer stronger, smarter, and more successful men.
2. Relationships: Nobody is going to love me the way I am.	Men have to initiate relationships. Other men are more effective than I.	Women can wait, pick and choose to accept relationship offers.
3. Needs: My needs will never be met if I have to rely on others.	Men have external power in jobs and money but will give in on issues to keep women happy.	Women make decisions at home and in other areas. They are impressed by money, possessions, and security.
4. Sexuality: Sex is my most important need.	Men are more sexual than women and freer to enjoy it. They will take sex whenever they can get it and cannot be trusted around women.	Women are less sexual than men and have to be coaxed into being sexual. Consequently, they are responsible for moral behaviors and can use sex as a reward or punishment.

7

CYBERSEX AND PORN
ADDICTION
WHAT IS CYBERSEX?

The most typical online/social media-driven sexual behaviors are listed below. NOTE that being involved with anyone or more than one of them, even on a regular basis, is not indicative of a problem, but when these experiences are abused to the point where they become all-consuming, interfering with day-to-day life, their abuse indicates evidence of a clear problem:

- Using social media sites to search for sexualized imagery and potential sex partners
- Sexting (the sending and receiving of explicit sexual images with or without masturbation)
- Seeking (or selling) sexual favors through websites such as Craigslist and Backpage, as well as more traditional dating and hookup websites and apps.
- Using websites and apps to find and connect with PNP (party and play) partners (drugs and sex)

- Looking for and participating in marathon sex or group sex with partners found through websites and apps.
- Webcam exhibitionism and voyeurism, which is common on chat sites that pair chat partners at random.
- Teledildonic masturbatory devices that warm, lubricate, pulse, and grip in tandem with onscreen sexual activities (such as porn videos or even via live webcam performances)
- Virtual-reality sex games in which users create customized fantasy avatars (animated selves) are then used to participate in interactive online sexcapades.
- Webcam, video, anime, prostitution, images, and other forms of online porn.

THE FACE OF PORNOGRAPHY ADDICTION

The Internet is rife with porn of every ilk imaginable, and people of every age, race, religion, gender, and sexual orientation are viewing it. Research suggests that approximately 12 percent of all websites offer pornographic content, and 35 percent of all downloads involve erotic content. To be honest, the amount of current (mostly free) online porn is increasing by the minute, owing primarily to user-generated imagery (sexts, webcam mutual masturbation sessions, etc.)

Furthermore, the barriers to accessing porn that once existed—cost, proof of age, etc.—are no more in existence. Today, all a person needs to do to get into porn is go to a porn site and start clicking. So it's hardly a surprise that porn addiction is among the most common forms of sex/cybersex addiction.

Many porn addicts couple their porn use with compulsive masturbation and various forms of non-intimate partner sex such as webcam sex, sexting, anonymous sex, casual sex, affairs, use of prostitutes, exhibitionism, voyeurism, etc. However, porn addiction is frequently a separate form of compulsive sexuality.

Porn addiction occurs when a person consistently loses control over whether or not he or she views and uses pornography, how much time he or she spends with pornography, and what types of pornography he or she uses. According to research, most porn addicts in today's world spend at least eleven or twelve hours per week looking at (and usually masturbating to) pornography, most of which is digital imagery accessed via their computer, laptop, tablet, smartphone, or other Internet-enabled devices! (While magazines, VHS tapes, DVDs, and other "traditional" forms of pornography are still used, the vast majority of porn addicts prefer the anonymity, affordability, and 24/7/365 accessibility that digital technologies provide.) And this eleven or twelve-hour-per-week figure is at the low end of the spectrum. Many porn addicts devote twice or even three times as much time to their addiction.

The following are common indicators that casual porn use has progressed to the level of addiction:

- Persistence of porn use despite consequences or promises made to self or others to stop
- Increasing amounts of time spent on porn

- Lost hours, if not days, searching for, viewing, and organizing pornography
- Excessive masturbation to the point of abrasion or injury
- Watching increasingly arousing, intense, or bizarre sexual content
- Lying about, concealing, or concealing the nature and extent of pornographic use
- Anger or irritability when told to stop using porn
- A lack of interest in real-world sex and relationship intimacy, if not a complete lack of interest.
- Sexual dysfunction in men (erectile dysfunction, delayed ejaculation, inability to reach orgasm)
- Feelings of loneliness, longing, and detachment that are deeply ingrained
- Drug/alcohol abuse combined with pornographic use
- Relapse of drug/alcohol addiction as a result of pornographic use or feelings about pornographic use
- With them, increased objectification of strangers was viewed as body parts rather than people.
- Progress from viewing two-dimensional images to using the Internet for casual/anonymous sexual hookups, paid sex, and so on.

Unfortunately, porn addicts are often hesitant to seek help because they do not see their hidden, often shameful solo sexual behaviors as the root cause of their unhappiness. When they seek help, it is often for addiction-related symptoms such as depression, loneliness, and relationship problems rather than the porn problem itself. Many people attend psychotherapy for long periods of time without ever discussing (or being asked about) pornography or masturbation. It's either too embarrassing for them to talk about it, or they don't see the connection between their porn use and the problems they're having in life. As a result, their primary issue remains hidden and unaddressed.

PORN-INDUCED SEXUAL DYSFUNCTION

As you may have noticed from the preceding list of possible implications of porn addiction, male porn addicts sometimes experience sexual dysfunction related to their porn abuse. In fact, erectile dysfunction (ED), delayed ejaculation (DE), and inability to reach orgasm (anorgasmia) are all increasingly documented consequences of pornography abuse. One 2012 survey of 350 self-identified sex addicts found that 26.7 percent reported issues with sexual dysfunction. Similar studies, smaller in scale, show comparable results. One such study, looking at twenty-four male sex addicts, found that one in six (16.7 percent) reported erectile dysfunction. Another, this one looking at nineteen male sex addicts, found that eleven of the nineteen (58 percent) reported some form of sexual dysfunction.

Put simply, growing numbers of physically healthy men, including men in their sexual prime, are suffering from sexual dysfunction—typically with real partners rather than with porn—and their dysfunction is directly related to their abuse of online pornography. Also, the frequency of masturbation and orgasm outside of a primary relationship is not entirely to blame for this issue (i.e., the need for a sexual refractory period during which males "reload," as it were). In fact, when a man spends 70%, 80%, or even 90% of his sexual life masturbating to online porn—endless photographs of sexy, thrilling, frequently changing partners and experiences—he is likely to find his real partner(s) less sexually satisfying than the visuals parading through his mind over time. As a result, the digital porn explosion has caused emotional/psychological disconnection in some men, which manifests physically as sexual dysfunction with real partners.

The following are some symptoms of porn-induced male sexual dysfunction:

- A man can achieve erections and orgasms through pornography, but he struggles with one or both when he's with a real-life partner.
- A man can have sex and experience orgasm with real-world partners, but it takes a long time, and his partners complain that he appears disengaged.
- A man can maintain an erection with real-world partners, but he can only achieve orgasm by replaying pornographic videos in his mind.
- A man prefers pornography to sex with a real partner because it is more intense and engaging.

The simple, sad truth is that, due to excessive porn consumption, an increasing number of men are suffering from sexual dysfunction, such as ED, DE, and anorgasmia. Worse still, not just men but also their intimate partners are affected by male sexual dysfunction. After all, if a man can't get it up, hold it up, or reach orgasm, it's possible that his partner's sexual satisfaction will suffer as well.

No Matter Where You Play, Sex Addiction Is Sex Addiction.

It is important to note that the fundamentals of sexual addiction are the same whether or not technology is involved. Simply put, cybersex addicts engage in problematic sexual behaviors on a consistent and compulsive basis, despite clearly related negative life consequences. As a result, their relationships (if they have them) are jeopardized, school and work become difficult, and they lose interest in recreation, hobbies, and other activities they once enjoyed.

Cybersex addicts also tend to isolate themselves, keep secrets, and lie to those close to them about their hypersexual behavior, often experiencing crippling shame about not only their behavior but also their lies and secrecy. Sometimes they make promises to themselves and others that they will stop their troubling behaviors, only to return to them a short time later. In these ways, the challenges of sexual addiction are the same as they have always been.

The fact that digital technology in today's world so

thoroughly facilitates sexually addictive fantasies and activities is simply a byproduct of the Internet era. In other words, the primary change in sexual addiction in recent years has been the ease and speed with which addicts can locate and access the sexual content and partners that fuel their addictions.

While sexnology undoubtedly facilitates and drives modern-day sexual addiction, it is also worth noting that it isn't entirely the cause of sexual addiction. In fact, as stated in the first paragraph of this section, most healthy people can use porn, hookup apps, and the like in a non-compulsive and life-affirming manner.

They do not become addicted, nor do they suffer negative consequences. People who are predisposed to anxiety, addiction, depression, compulsivity, impulsivity, and other mental health issues can struggle with sexnology in the same way they struggle with alcohol, narcotics, gambling, or any other potentially addictive substance or behavior. As a result, the increasing availability of digitized sexual content and partners does not increase the likelihood that these people will struggle in life; it merely increases the likelihood that their struggles will be sexual in nature.

8

THE PORN MYTH: THE REALITY BEHIND THE FANTASY OF PORNOGRAPHY

I have too many romantic fantasies, and they make
me sad.
— Graham Coxon, Author: *Superstate*

1. PORN IS JUST "ADULT" ENTERTAINMENT

Pornographers are fond of saying that pornography is
sophisticated entertainment for mature adults. Porn,
they'll have you believe, are something only mature people
enjoy.

2. TO BE ANTI-PORN IS TO BE ANTI-SEX.

Saying that we need porn to avoid sexual repression is
like saying that we need gluttony to avoid anorexia.
Pornography is a celebration of sex in the same way that
gluttony is a celebration of food. In both cases, what
should be appreciated is twisted into something unhealthy

and dangerous rather than being appreciated at all. We gorge the masses on industrialized, commodified sexuality by putting sex—any kind of sex—into the medium of pornography. This in no way celebrates sex. It devalues it.

At its core, modern pornography is an industry. It is about the commodification of bodies for revenue. And it is precisely because I'm for sex that I'm against porn. Whether we're talking about misogynist women-hating porn or the gentle girl-on-girl variety, it is pornography as a medium that is the main problem. Porn is the business of presenting women's bodies to men for masturbation. To stand against this is not to stand against sex generally but to stand against a habit of solo sex that turns men into consumers, not lovers.

3. THERE IS NO DIFFERENCE BETWEEN PORN AND NAKED ART.

Pornographers often speak of their work as being in the cultural continuum of erotic art. Porn has been around since the beginning of time, they say, and will never go away. They appeal to antiquity, noting that some of the most celebrated works of classic art feature nudity. The Renaissance celebrated this heritage; thus, Michelangelo's David is nude, and so are many of his painted figures in the Sistine Chapel.

So, what exactly is the distinction between pornography and naked art? First and foremost, their definitions differ. The term "pornography" is derived from the Greek root porne, which means "prostitution" or "prostitute." Pornography, like prostitution, has a specific goal in mind:

sexual stimulation in order to produce a completed sexual act. True art is not created to serve as a substitute for a prostitute. True artists aim at capturing their vision of beauty so that the beautiful might be apprehended and appreciated.

A porn director would be puzzled or even disappointed if someone who watched one of his X-rated flicks told him, "The film was beautiful, but it didn't get me off; I didn't find it all that sexually arousing." On the other hand, Michelangelo would most likely have been disturbed if someone told him that his paintings in the Sistine Chapel did little to arouse wonder but sure did turn him on. The difference between a pornographer and an artist lies in his intentions.

No doubt, the line between pornography and art can be blurry. Some say that the artistic value of porn is in the eye of the beholder. Perhaps it is. But, in the end, porn isn't made for the sake of beauty, and true art isn't made for the sake of masturbation.

4. ONLY RELIGIOUS PEOPLE OPPOSE PORN.

A couple of matters should be made clear at the outset. First, just because some people oppose porn because it violates the morality taught by their religion does not mean their cause is wrong. During the nineteenth-century movement to abolish slavery, many Quakers opposed the trans-Atlantic slave trade because it violated their religion's precepts, which teaches equality. Their religious motivation did not make their cause wrong.

Second, in a free society, people should not be

excluded from civil discourse or be discounted as having nothing to contribute to it just because they accept the morals taught by their religion. Many people who are against stealing and murder were taught the Ten Commandments in their churches or synagogues. Should their upbringing exclude them from public discussions about violent crime?

Now that we've gotten those out of the way, we can get down to business with the myth. Is it true that only religious people condemn pornography?

Several years ago, the magazine GQ ran a thought-provoking article about why men should quit looking at porn. The same year that GQ dished out provocative photos of the hundred "sexiest women of the twenty-first century," the magazine also told their readers that masturbating to images of sexy women might be a bad idea. What spurred this advice? Editors of the magazine had stumbled upon a growing group on Reddit.com called NoFap, an online community of (mostly) men who were challenging each other to put away porn and masturbation.

This community began not because of religious motivations but because its members wanted to see how quitting porn and masturbation would improve their overall health and well-being. About 64 percent of NoFappers had developed tastes for porn that had become extreme or deviant. Among the twenty-seven- to thirty-one-year-olds in the group, 19 percent were suffering from premature ejaculation, 25 percent were totally disinterested in sex with a partner, 31 percent had difficulty reaching orgasm, and 34 percent were experiencing erectile dysfunction. After joining the NoFap community and quitting their porn habits, 60 percent found that their sexual function improved.

In an interview with the NoFap community founder, Alexander Rhodes, he described himself as an agnostic. At the time of the interview, most NoFappers considered themselves atheists or agnostics, and currently, there are well over 150,000 online members. When asked why he started the community, Rhodes said, "Love is my motivation." He wants to see people live porn-free lives because he honestly believes we are better off without it. Comparing pornography to cigarettes, he said, "It is always a harmful thing to consume."

Men like Rhodes and the thousands of nonreligious individuals in his online community are not alone in their disdain for pornography. Men with damaged libidos are not the only ones who think pornography is a problem; thousands of women do as well. In the 1960s, '70s, and '80s, the world saw the rise of a new wave of feminists who ardently spoke out against the social ills of pornography— and these same women often also opposed organized religion.

In conclusion, religious people are not the only ones who oppose porn. There are others who oppose it because personal experience, social science, or medical research has shown that porn is not conducive to their well-being.

5. WOMEN DON'T STRUGGLE WITH PORN.

Pornography is typically seen as something that men do: men create it; men watch it; men get addicted to it. Women are often seen as the victims of pornography.

Pornography objectifies women; it abuses them and teaches men to abuse them. Those are the common story-lines. Men are the aggressors, taught by a poor teacher, and women suffer because of it.

If a woman watches pornography, it is usually assumed that her boyfriend or husband wants her to watch it with him. A recent study of heterosexual women who used porn concluded: "This suggests that when heterosexual women consume pornography, they usually do it in the company of their partner."

Some of these women watching porn may be doing so under pressure from their partners. What we often fail to discuss, however, is the fact that some women watch pornography of their own accord, and some of those women feel they simply cannot stop.

While pornography use among women is rarely discussed, it is on the rise. One study indicated that 50 percent of female adolescents had used pornography in the previous six months. Other studies indicate that 25 percent of women ages eighteen to thirty-four use pornography. Even 4 percent of women ages fifty to sixty-five admit to using pornography. These statistics include any type of porn use, from occasional to frequent. About 2 percent of women use pornography multiple times per week.

In contrast to those numbers, during a Pew Research Center study conducted in 2010, only 2 percent of the women surveyed admitted to watching pornography online. In 2013, that number jumped to 8 percent. If other studies are to be believed, that number is actually much higher.

While the research about pornography use among women varies, statistics from porn websites themselves don't lie. According to statistics from 2014, gathered by one of the top-ranking porn sites in the world, 23 percent of their viewers are women, nearly one woman for every five men. In America, females currently make up 15 percent of the viewing population.

The common perception has been that men are more prone than women to watch pornography because they are more visually wired; therefore, they find sexual images more arousing. On the other hand, women have been assumed to be more emotionally and relationally wired and therefore less aroused by mere images. When women turn to sexual material, it has been thought, they are more likely to reach for a romance novel or erotica than for pornography. However, some studies have shown that women can be just as aroused by pornography as men are.

When compared with the stimulation from nonsexual images, pornographic images create two to three times the response in the brain—for men and women.

6. NOT MASTURBATING IS UNHEALTHY FOR A GUY.

Perhaps no one has had a more profound impact on modern sexual ideas and morals than Sigmund Freud. The modern rejection of the notion that masturbation is a misuse of one's sexual powers can be traced to him. "It has appeared to me that masturbation is the one great habit that is a 'primary addiction,'" Freud wrote, "and that the other addictions, such as alcohol, morphine, tobacco, excessive gambling, and so on, only enter life as a substitute and replacement for it." For many men, masturbation is as natural to their lives as urination. It is a biological need that fulfills an important function—and a pleasurable one, at that.

But masturbation has long been a taboo. In 1760, the Swiss physician Samuel Auguste Tissot published his now-famous L'Onanismo, his dissertation on the physical ailments produced by masturbation. He believed that masturbating too much could lead to blurred vision, headaches, memory loss, gout, rheumatic disorders, and other medical problems.

At this point, some clarity is needed. No doctor claims that masturbation will make you go blind and crazy, but neither should we claim, as some do, that avoiding masturbation is unhealthy. After all, when medical professionals say that masturbation is healthy for you, they aren't talking about getting your heart rate up and your circulation moving, which can be accomplished in other ways.

When some claim that masturbation is healthy, they are talking about ejaculation. Take prostate cancer, for instance. When Santella and Cooper claim that frequent masturbation lowers the risk of prostate cancer, they cite a mixed-result analysis published in the Journal of the American Medical Association.

Researchers write, "Nine studies observed a statistically significant or non-significant positive association; 3 studies reported no association; 7 studies found a statistically significant or non-significant inverse relationship, and 1 study found a U-shaped relationship." What does that mean in layman's terms? Ejaculation frequency is not related to prostate cancer.

This should hardly surprise us. Sex is necessary for the survival and the flourishing of the human race, so it makes sense that sexual intercourse would come with some positive side effects.

If ejaculations are healthy, you might assume that those caused by masturbation are too, but they aren't. No one knows why exactly. The male body simply responds differently in different instances of ejaculation. Even the makeup of semen is different when ejaculations from masturbation and vaginal intercourse are compared.

Modern studies have found that frequent masturbation is associated with:

- More prostate abnormalities
- Less ability to recover from erectile dysfunction
- Less satisfaction with one's mental health
- Less relationship satisfaction
- Depression and less happiness

The fact is this: there is no documented health problem associated with refraining from masturbation, and the jury is still out on whether the practice has demonstrable positive health effects from the act.

However, putting the health question aside, we can get to the heart of why men masturbate in the first place. After all, no one ever masturbated while fantasizing about reduced cancer risks.

We live in a society where it is so normal to escape into a world of sexual fantasy that we hardly believe there could be another way of living. But this isn't a universal human experience. The Aka people, for instance, are a traditional hunter-gatherer tribe in the Central African Republic. They forage for edible plants, set up encampments in the rain forests, and engage in ritual dances and elaborate polyphonic songs. To Westerners, their ways may seem bizarre, mysterious, or even strangely beautiful. They also don't have a word in their language for "masturbation." It is simply not part of their cultural model of sexuality.

Contrast this with men in Western society: 25 percent of adult men say they masturbate daily or several times a week; 55 percent say they masturbate daily to monthly, and about half of boys, fourteen to seventeen years old, masturbate at least twice a week. Escaping into sexual fantasy is the norm.

What is the impact of this lifestyle of fantasy, this habit of escaping into a mental world of sexual pleasure? In a letter to a friend, Oxford scholar C. S. Lewis offered some insights about masturbation. He said that a man's sexual appetite is meant to lead him out of himself, lead him into being a self-gift that completes and corrects his personality—first by sharing whole-life oneness with a lover, second by procreating children. On the other hand, masturbation "sends the man back into the jail of himself, there to hold a harem of fantasy brides."

What's the harm in doing this? According to Lewis, the problem with masturbation is that it causes a man to prefer his fantasy world to reality. In the end, they're just a conduit for him to adore himself more and more. After all, almost the whole point of life is to break free from ourselves, from the small dark prisons into which we are all born. Masturbation, like anything else that slows down the recovery process, should be avoided. The danger is falling in love with the prison.

7. PORN PREVENTS RAPE AND SEXUAL VIOLENCE.

For some, this makes intuitive sense. If you are the kind of man who wants to rape a woman, perhaps sitting at home and masturbating to porn more or less gets it out of your system. It should be stated right away: the argument that porn causes all men to commit violent sex crimes is clearly false, and no serious critic of pornography would make such a claim. More men consume porn now than ever before, and yet most porn-watching men would shudder at the thought of violently raping a woman. Pornography is not a sufficient or necessary condition for rape.

There are, however, several reasons why we should be skeptical of the idea that porn actually prevents sexual violence.

- First, a supposed decline in rape can also be correlated to other factors, such as more education about rape and sexual violence or greater measures of protection for women.
- Second, the National Crime Victimization Survey (NCVS) claims that rape prevalence is rapidly declining based on inadequate data collection. The National Violence Against Women Study, the National College Women Sexual Victimization Study, and The National

Women's Study all report higher rape and sexual assault rates than the NCVS. The National Research Council has found multiple problems with the ways rape data has been collected by the NCVS. Rape and sexual assault are, unfortunately, grossly underreported.

8. PORN ISN'T ADDICTIVE.

The concept of "sex addiction" has been around for a long time. Sigmund Freud considered masturbation the original addiction—something common to us all—and that all other addictions were a substitute or replacement for it.

Many, however, doubt that sex or porn can truly be addictive. Sexual pleasure is, after all, as natural as the day is long. Sex is not something we inject into our veins or snort up our noses. People may use sex in unhealthy ways, but sex addiction, they claim, is total fiction.

True, not everyone who cheats on their spouse should use the label "sex addict" as an excuse—what is often labeled an addiction is just a person's selfishness. It is also correct that there are often other underlying issues that drive someone's unhealthy sexual habits. However, writing off the idea that sex can be addictive is completely wrong.

In order to understand why sex can become an addiction, one first needs to understand why things like drugs are addictive. The very reason drugs are addictive at all is because they "trick" the brain: they activate the brain's natural neural pathways, which are involved in reinforcement and pleasure. Pornography activates powerful neurotransmitters such as epinephrine (also known as adrenaline), dopamine, and others, making it addictive when used compulsively.

Sex and porn addictions are realities, and just as with alcoholism or drug addiction, the label "addict" does not excuse a person for his actions. Addiction is slavery, to be sure, but it is a chosen slavery. Addicts find freedom not by denying the power that porn has over them, not by denying that their addiction is real, but by admitting it to others and asking for help.

9. PORN IS ONLY FANTASY: IT DOESN'T AFFECT OUR REAL LIVES.

Although most pornography is scripted and heavily edited, this does not diminish its impact on the viewer, his body, and his relationships. To comprehend the full extent of pornography's ability to influence our sexual behavior, we must first comprehend how the human mind learns. Humans participate in a process known as observational learning. We learn how to do something by watching someone else do it.

Online porn viewing is, among other things, novelty-seeking behavior: constantly clicking, greedily keeping multiple tabs open, and always looking for the next girl, the next sexual buzz. A real woman—no matter how attractive—is only one woman. A man this obsessed will have difficulty finding her arousing.

Can the fantasy of pornography have an impact on our daily lives? The answer is unequivocally yes.

10. MARRIED LIFE WILL CURE US OF OUR PORN OBSESSIONS.

Many single men and women hooked on porn will say, "Once I get married, this won't be a problem anymore." They think that once they have a readily available sexual partner, porn will lose its pull. Maybe they think that being committed to someone will be a strong enough motivation to kick the habit. This expectation shows a failure to understand what an obsession with porn really is.

Married life no more cures a porn addiction than winning the lottery cures a gambling addiction. A person so trained on the pornographic experience isn't merely after a good orgasm. He is addicted to the rush of moving from one object of desire to the next, one body to the next, always looking to trade the one in front of his eyes for what he believes to be the ultimate sexual experience.

Unless there is deep change, a person hooked on this kind of experience will not be cured by marriage. Instead, the porn obsession just might destroy the marriage.

As mentioned before, thinking that marriage will cure a porn addiction is a bit like thinking that money will cure gambling addiction. In gambling, the addiction is not to the money but to the high that results from chasing the money. Giving a gambling addict money only fuels the habit because he is addicted to the feeling that gambling gives him.

While not yet officially described as addictive, pornography use triggers the same centers in the brain as drug abuse, gambling, and other behaviors that can become compulsive. Porn addicts are hooked on the high they get from chasing after sexual fantasies. The unrealistic expectations that are fed by porn are what carry over into and destroy relationships because no person can live up to the on-demand, anything-goes sex depicted in movies. When faced with the inevitable difficulties of establishing and maintaining a human relationship, it is much easier for a porn addict to opt for the instant relief of virtual sex. Marriage will not cure a pornographic habit, but a pornographic habit will almost certainly destroy a marriage.

9

HOW PORN REWIRES YOUR BRAIN

When you watch porn, your brain thinks you are having sex. Horniness is the evolutionary drive that pushes you to do whatever is necessary to have sex and make babies. Your brain can't comprehend the difference between watching a video and having real sex. Your brain's mirror neurons visualize you doing the same thing, and a part of your brain responds as if you were. It's kind of like how when watching a scary movie, we cringe or jump out of our seats. Or a sad movie can make you cry and feel sad. The brain thinks something that you watch digitally is actually happening to you in real life, and it acts accordingly. If you're watching multiple porn scenes (which is usually the case for most porn binges), your brain thinks you are having sex with multiple partners.

To sum it up, all this sex overstimulates your brain, which desensitizes it, causes problems in your sex life, and reduces your ability to enjoy life.

Let's break this down. Dopamine is a brain chemical that motivates you to do something that your brain thinks will make it feel good, like having sex or eating food. Our brain makes us experience pleasure when we engage in these life-giving and enjoyable activities, which have kept humans alive for millions of years.

Your brain uses dopamine, a neurochemical, to train you to recognize good and bad activities. When you do actions that your brain says are good for survival, it rewards you with a shot of dopamine that triggers the sensation of pleasure and stimulates memory and concentration. It creates arousal and excitement just before you have sex, pushing you to complete what you started.

For instance, think of a Thanksgiving dinner where you starved yourself all day, and finally, your aunt said, "Okay, it's ready, everyone grab a plate!" And remember that sensation as you rushed to the kitchen to fill up your plate. You sat down and shoved endless amounts of food into your mouth without even chewing because you were so excited. That intense rush? Yes, that's dopamine.

Imagine seeing a woman walking right by you who appeared to be the most beautiful woman you had ever seen, and you felt a rush of both nervousness and excitement. Yes, that's dopamine too. Or think about when you had a new business idea that you believed would change an industry, and you were the first one ever to think of it... yeah, that's just dopamine.

Now that we understand what dopamine is and how it makes you feel, the question remains: How does it relate to porn?

The problem with porn is that it gives off a massive shot of dopamine to your brain. It's too much dopamine for your brain to handle at once because your brain was never designed to handle unlimited amounts of porn of highly attractive women with enlarged breasts and perfect to hip-weight ratios. It's simply unreal and too good for your brain to handle.

As you're watching porn, the dopamine rush encourages you to masturbate to produce even more dopamine. Simultaneously, you release even more happy chemicals in your brain like serotonin and dopamine, which end in an orgasm. Why would anyone not enjoy this?

It's easy, it feels good, and it's free... and that's exactly the problem. Sexual arousal is nature's number one priority driven by dopamine. Your brain starts to crave more and more, causing you to watch more and more porn.

Sexual stimulation and orgasm give our brains' reward systems the biggest natural shot of dopamine of all. This makes sense. That big dopamine shot from an orgasm then goes on to wire our brain's reward system to encourage us to repeat whatever behavior we did to get sex so we can continue to get sex in the future.

But the problem is you're not having sex at all, and your brain cannot differentiate the difference between porn and real sex. It thinks you're winning in life when you're watching porn, so it's reacting as it should. Don't blame your brain. Your brain thinks you're mating with real women, so it encourages you to go do whatever you just did to get that stimulus again since it's wired to do that.

Pay attention; this is when it gets even more dangerous. The Internet gives you an unlimited variety of sexual experiences. When viewed, this variety means that dopamine shoots to your brain, training you to search for more and more porn.

And what you once found arousing over time will no longer be arousing. You develop a level of tolerance to past experiences. So you search for different types of novel porn such as anal, gangbang, incest, teen, cartoon porn, and so on to give you that same level of dopamine rush you now need to ejaculate.

This tolerance can take years to develop, but it's very easy to develop since the pleasure reward system of your brain loves watching porn, masturbating, and orgasms.

Neurons firing and wiring together are also how our habits are formed. When you receive a shot of dopamine after receiving some reward – whether food, sex, or novelty – your brain strengthens the neurons that fired and wired together to achieve the reward so that you will repeat the process and can get it again in the future. The rewiring involves connecting the cues and behavior that led to a pleasurable reward.

This cue behavior reward connection is what author Charles Duhigg calls The Habit Loop. Cues cause dopamine to release, such as sitting at a computer alone late at night. Or it means surfing Instagram or some other social media outlets where you see half-naked women. Or cues to watch porn come when you're just feeling a little depressed, bored, distracted, or stressed.

Repeat this circuit for a few days or weeks, and you've got a connection that leads to you checking out porn without even thinking about it – and worse, you can't control it. It can become difficult to control because it's now wired into your brain. Porn surfing simply becomes a habit.

Throughout most of your brain's evolution, sex was a limited commodity, and it was a good survival strategy to look for sex whenever possible. Now that you have access to an infinite amount of sex online, this is no longer a good strategy.

Too much sexual stimulation has health risks of its own, like reduced sensitivity to dopamine, which reduces the enjoyment of activities you once found pleasurable.

The only way for you to feel "good" again is to continue watching heavier and heavier scenes of porn such as gangbangs, abuse, incest, and double penetration, which sends you into a downward spiral of porn addiction.

PORN IS MORE DANGEROUS THAN COCAINE AND HEROIN

Speaking before the U.S. Senate in 2004, Dr Jeffrey Satinover stated, "Modern science enables us to comprehend that the underlying nature of a pornographic addiction is chemically identical to a heroin addiction." Cocaine and heroin provide an instant rush of dopamine to your brain, giving you that euphoric feel-good effect. So does porn.

But porn is more dangerous than cocaine and heroin because, unlike most addictive behaviors such as alcohol, drugs, and gambling, porn has no barriers.

Psychologists and addiction experts have found that if an addiction meets fewer and fewer of what is known as the three 'As' of addiction, it's easier to become an addict:

- Accessibility
- Affordability
- Anonymity

Like alcohol or drug addictions, most addictions will have one or two of those. But the cost is often the biggest barrier for most addicts. But what is astounding is that porn meets all three conditions:

Accessibility: You can go online and watch unlimited amounts of porn within seconds.

Affordability: It's free.

Anonymity: It's on your phone or computer, and no one will ever know.

Knowing this can help you understand why porn is so dangerous. The environment for a porn user to become an addict is the easiest of all known addictions in the world.

Your brain views sex as a top priority, not alcohol, drugs, or gambling. When you give a porn user unending novelty for free, he will abuse it, not because something is wrong with him but because it's wired into his DNA.

And since your brain cannot differentiate the difference between porn and real sex, then the porn user is only doing what he is supposed to do. It's not his fault that he is aroused by porn and watches dozens of scenes.

Let's take this example, for instance. The main barriers of alcohol are the age limit, the cost, and the hangover. What if at any age, with the press of one button, you could order an endless amount of alcohol to your house, no one would ever know how much you drank, and the next day you would have no hangover?

Yes, in that case, we would all be alcoholics. Now

imagine a world where every type of alcohol was free, and no matter how much you drank, it cost you nothing... This is the world of porn, where there is no (enforced) age limit, it is free, and no one will ever know if you watched it.

Psychologists say addictive behaviors will meet some barriers. We've already discussed cost. But there's also the barrier of privacy. If you drank a bottle of whiskey before or during work, then people would know something was wrong with you, and you'd get caught.

Yet if you watch porn, no one will ever know, and surprisingly the porn usage is mostly done on mobile devices; why? Because it's typically viewed in the privacy of your room. I bet your friends and family have gone years without ever knowing that you've been watching porn and that you may have a problem with it.

Because the barriers are so low and a free-for-all online, there's the perfect environment for an addiction to develop. Let's get this clear: Porn is a sexual stimulant, and it's the most dangerous kind of stimulant in the world.

Porn use and drug use have a lot in common. When cocaine users escalate their behavior, they need bigger and more frequent hits of cocaine. When porn users escalate their behavior, they need more extreme porn more frequently. You need a bigger dose to keep generating the same dopamine reward.

In practice, porn sessions become longer and more frequent. Your brain tries to make up in quantity for what it can't get in quality. An extreme user may spend hours each day watching porn.

Eventually, it can get weird and taboo to become something violent, disgusting, dangerous, or illegal. Or possibly it gets to the point where a man goes off the computer and starts to engage in strip clubs, prostitutes, and illegal sex work.

Violent material can feature degradation, verbal abuse, rape scenes, and serious physical and traumatic injuries to women. Disgusting material can feature incest porn, sex with animals, urine, feces, or anything objectionable that will produce the desired effect. Dangerous material is anything where you or the performer would be in trouble if caught, such as material with underage girls or sneaky pictures or a video you took without the person's consent.

This level of porn usage can take years to develop– it's not something that happens overnight. But if you look back at your porn use, you may see that it slowly started with casual sex, then moved on to anal, and then turned into more violent, disgusting, or dangerous scenes.

Next time you watch a porn scene that you like, consider how extreme it is in violence, disgusting elements, and danger. Did you always like this kind of scene, or would you have found it too extreme earlier in your life?

Let's now go into the different types of porn users and see where you currently fit.

10

THE THREE TYPES OF PORN USERS

The three different types and stages of porn use are the casual users, the at-risk user, and the addict. The casual user watches porn for fun. It's an occasional distraction depending on life circumstances but not too extreme, nor does it block out important activities.

It's more of an enjoyable distraction, a sporadic form of escape or relaxation that is NOT as satisfying or meaningful as real intimate connections. The frequency of use is driven by life-changing events.

For the casual user, there is no history of neglect or abuse. Porn and online sexual experiences are not sustained because they feel unrealistic, and he'd rather pursue real relationships with women. He doesn't experience any shame or high levels of guilt after watching porn.

An at-risk user will have periods of intense engagement, and it is a distraction from other life challenges. But he does know how to limit it or stop when he starts to experience more serious consequences.

The at-risk user will typically keep it as a secret in

exchange for looking good or being accepted, although he may have a potential history of abuse for recreation, spending, gambling, sex, and other high-intensity behaviors as a result of reacting to life stressors. The main difference that makes an at-risk user different from an addict is that the at-risk user has the ability to stop when he sees it's becoming a problem. An addict has lost the ability to choose to stop.

Addicts turn to digital sexual fantasies to fill an emotional void. They cannot stop negative behaviors even when they are not helping their life or even have a desire for change.

They know what they're doing is hurting them, yet they still keep doing it. They typically are depressed or are experiencing severe emotional challenges or have a history of substance abuse, childhood abuse, neglect, family dysfunction, addiction, mental illness, and lifelong fears of being unwanted or "not enough," so they use porn and masturbation to replace intimate personal relationships and peer support altogether.

There could also be a history of unresolved adult trauma, having infrequent short-term relationships, and being emotionally distant from friendships and family even if they are physically in close proximity.

Addicts find as much intensity, excitement, and distraction in searching for the next sexual thrill as in the sex act itself. Fantasies pull addicts into an emotional state that renders them unable to make better choices or even consider how their behaviors might affect others or themselves.

Questions to ask yourself:

- Do you find yourself spending an increasing amount of time online watching porn and engaging in sexual or romantic fantasies, despite the fact that you have more important things to do in your life?
- Have you promised yourself that you would stop viewing certain porn websites or using apps and find yourself back there again?
- Do you collect porn?
- Have you experienced negative consequences in relationships, at school, work, or in other important areas of your life due to your porn use?
- Has your porn use led to a reduction in friends, family, recreational activities?
- Has your porn use caused you to lose anything or anyone important to you?
- Do you lie or keep secrets about your porn use?
- Do you hide your porn use so others won't discover it?
- Do you feel like your porn use interferes with personal goals, relationships, and healthy intimacy?
- Do you become defensive or extremely ashamed when you look at porn?

I want this to be a slap in the face for you if you responded yes to all of the above questions. Get up! If you continue on this course, it will only be a matter of time before you advance from your current stage to the next. So you may be wondering if it is possible to become addicted to porn.

Yes, addiction is a compulsion to continue self-destructive habits despite serious consequences with an inability to control cravings. Sexual behavior addictions are as real as drug addictions, according to the American Society of Addiction Medicine's new definition of addiction (August 2011).

Yourbrainonporn.com compared Internet porn to excessive gambling, video game playing, and food addiction, all of which can cause brain changes that mimic drug addiction.

Here are three signs an addiction is developing:

- Sexual obsession where you spend a large amount of time thinking, planning, or doing the actual activity.
- Loss of control where the behavior has become compulsive, and the person has lost the ability to stop when he or she wishes.
- Negative consequences are developing such as relationship problems, education, physical or emotional, social anxiety, depression, apathy, brain fog, loss of interest in previously enjoyable activities, and potential legal troubles.

Whatever actions you do daily, whether good or bad, will become a part of who you are and have associated consequences. Porn addicts spend on average 11 hours per week engaging in porn – on some weeks, it's double that. It becomes an addiction when someone loses control and can't limit porn viewing and when they move to alternative genres of porn to get the same type of stimulation they received in the past.

Using porn was all about having a good time, escaping worries and pleasures, and getting a chance to do things one couldn't do in real life. Yet, most men don't stop to think that what they are doing is slowly becoming a habit and a daily ritual. Over time, men develop a relationship with porn, and porn easily slips into the role of 'significant other.' In this case, a man can be intimate or in a relationship with other women, but porn is what he truly desires and obsesses about.

And as the porn addiction develops, men find themselves easily becoming irritated and depressed, isolating from other people, sexually objectifying people, neglecting important areas of life, having problems with sex in real life, constantly feeling bad about themselves, and engaging in risky behaviors (like strip clubs, paying for sex, meeting up with strangers met online and so on).

Given a negative environment, it then becomes easier to go deeper and deeper into the realms of porn, thus sending the user into a downward spiral in life. In all, porn addiction is very real, and the consequences are very serious. According to a Native American legend, every person contains two wolves: one bad and one good. Which one will triumph, you may wonder? It's the one you feed.

❧ 11 ❧

WHY IT'S SO HARD TO STOP
WATCHING PORN

Scientists recently showed that methamphetamine and cocaine hijack the same reward center nerve cells that evolved for sexual conditioning. Simply put, addictive drugs like meth and cocaine are appealing because they exploit the very mechanisms that evolved to make sex appealing. And guess what, so can porn.

Sexual arousal is nature's top priority and raises dopamine the highest of all-natural rewards. Your brain starts to crave and then loses control, and negative consequences soon follow.

We're more inclined to be addicted to food and sex than we are to alcohol and drugs because nature wired humans this way. Humans can survive without alcohol and drugs but not sex and food.

Experts at Germany's Max Planck Institute discovered that more porn use was associated with less grey matter and reduced reward activity when viewing porn in the study "Brain Structure and Functional Connectivity Associated with Pornography Consumption" published in the Psychiatry Journal.

In other words, porn use weakens the prefrontal cortex, which reduces willpower so that you can easily succumb to more porn use and other addictive behaviors. This makes it easier to give up on other goals in life. Understand how dopamine works, and you understand why you are attracted to porn.

Porn acts as a substitute for actual sex, but your brain doesn't know that. It reacts to a picture or video of a naked woman the same way it does to a real-life naked woman or real sex. Your brain ramps up dopamine levels, driving you to orgasm whether that climax is fostered with another human being or is self-induced through masturbation.

Dopamine explains why certain types of porn are more compelling than others, and how in extreme cases, men prefer porn to actual sex.

When looking at a pornographic image, the brain becomes habituated to that stimulus, simply injecting more novelty and getting more dopamine. A porn video is more intense because the live-action activates your mirror neurons, making you feel like you're the one having sex.

The stronger the stimulation, the bigger the shot of dopamine to the reward system, which means the greater desire to watch that porn video. Porn offers the sexual novelty that dopamine has hardwired you to seek. The more you find new sexual experiences, the more dopamine you get, which reinforces the desire to look for even more sexual novelty. Porn's easy access to new experiences is the main reason why it is so hard to stop watching porn.

Men also receive a shot of dopamine whenever they encounter a new attractive woman other than their current partner. Their brains are hardwired to seek out as many different (novel) sexual partners as possible. Males are biologically driven to reproduce with as many different females as possible to create as many babies as possible, with as much genetic variation as possible to increase their possible bloodlines.

Men have a constant need for something new. For example, studies show that if you put a male rat in a cage with a female rat very quickly, he'll start having sex with the female rat. But after a while, he'll slowly reduce the frequency of sex and then eventually stop.

The moment you put a new female rat in the cage, the male rat will begin having sex with the female, and then slowly, the same thing will happen again. This leads to less and less sex over time and then eventually no sex at all. This trend will go on and on even if the male rat is tired or is starting to hurt himself with too much sex.

The drive for multiple new sex partners provides an extra burst of energy and arousal with each novel partner – even when you already have an available and willing one known as the Coolidge Effect. The effect happens in all mammalian brains (although in male brains slightly more than females). The Coolidge Effect is the key to why porn is so exciting and addicting.

With porn, you have access to new women with one click, for free and, no one will ever know. Every time you indulge in porn, your brain thinks you've found the evolutionary goldmine that stimulates your brain to keep on consuming more and more porn despite not knowing that you are watching a video.

Binging brings an evolutionary advantage. Thousands of years ago, if you found a berry plant, then you'd eat the entire plant since you would likely never find another anytime soon. Now with porn, it's like a mating season, yet it is a 24/7 mating season that never ends due to the unlimited availability of porn. The evolutionary advantage of binging is now a disadvantage. Porn is the junk food of sex except that the junk food is free and in your pocket 24/7.

Sex was a limited commodity throughout most of your brain's evolution, and it was a good survival strategy to go for sex whenever possible. Now that you have access to an infinite amount of sex online, this is no longer a good strategy. Too much sexual stimulation has health risks of its own: reduced sensitivity to dopamine, which reduces your overall quality of life.

The brain releases a level of neurochemicals that your brain can't handle and was never designed to handle. It's an artificial, supercharged response to a natural urge to have sex. Novelty is an extremely powerful desire – look at how humans always want what's new: the new video game, the new movie, the new TV series, the new restaurant, the new shoes. This is why it's so hard to stop watching porn because we constantly want more new scenes, and they are widely available for free.

Porn used to have barriers such as ordering it to your doorstep or going to the sketchy adult video store, peep shows, or an adult movie theatre. Men felt like they were "creepy" for engaging in these acts, but now with the advent of high-speed Internet and mobile capability, porn is in your pocket 100% of your day.

Porn's power to produce experiences of excitement, relaxation, and escape from pain makes it highly addictive. Over time, you may come to rely on it to make you feel good, and you may even require it to keep you from feeling bad. Cravings, preoccupations, and out-of-control behavior are common side effects of using it.

Pornography has the potential to be both your greatest need and your greatest liability. The more pornography a man watches, the less control he has over his thoughts and actions. He becomes enslaved by porn because he has rewired his brain to consume more and more porn. To put it bluntly, when you cannot let go of what controls you, you have become less human, not more.

Critical Questions:

- What problems has porn caused me in the past?
- What problems am I experiencing today because of my porn use?
- How has porn changed me in ways I don't like?
- How does my porn use hurt my intimate partner and others I care about?
- What problems might I face in the future if I keep watching porn?

THE SOCIAL PORN

Porn is anything that induces erotic thought. Although we often think of porn as hardcore penetration material, it can even be Playboy, Cosmopolitan, Maxim magazine,

Victoria's Secret brochure, or even that girl you follow on social media who's always half-naked...

Porn is all around us, and we live in a hyper-sexual world today because, well, sex sells, and the corporate giants are well aware of this.

The current reality seems to be getting worse every year as men are forming relationships with webcam girls, following girls they've never met on Instagram and other social media platforms. These aren't real relationships, and you're simply wasting your time following them.

Social porn is the gateway to hardcore porn online. If girls you follow on social media such as Facebook, Instagram, Snapchat pose half-naked, the image induces erotic thoughts. That's essentially porn.

Instagram girls you follow post hot photo after hot photo, always containing breasts, butt, or both. A hit of novelty comes if she's with her friends. These social media platforms are basically another avenue for a guy to view porn. You click and enlarge an erotic photo, and then you quickly scour through her entire portfolio of photos looking for another photo where hopefully she's revealing even more of her body. Why are you following these women anyways? Don't you have anything more important to do than stare in "awe" at these women who will never speak to you or give you their time? Instead of looking at women you wish you could be with, why don't you become the type of man that she would want to be with?

If there were no women on social media platforms, I am convinced these platforms would not be billion-dollar companies. They would simply be two guys in a garage with a piece of code.

Social porn is the perfect trigger to watching hardcore porn online since your mind is already thinking erotic thoughts. And all you have to do is click over, open a new tab, and in less than five seconds, you'll have unrestricted access to beautiful women doing whatever you want.

Stop finding pleasure in looking at other people's lives and being a spectator in this world and get to work on creating the life you truly want. You can start now and be in an entirely different place in just a few years, or you can stay the same. The choice is yours because if you don't ... well, let's get into that right now...

DESENSITIZATION TO REAL-LIFE

Porn addiction steals joy from other areas of your life since it impacts the value you get from rewards. And it becomes increasingly difficult to enjoy things that you once enjoyed.

To better understand this idea, think about this: Your brain transfers dopamine along paths of linked nerve cells. Normally this dopamine moves from one to the next without any problems, leading to a positive experience.

It's released by the sending cell and picked up by the receiving cell's dopamine receptors. But when on porn, your brain is overstimulated, and the sending cell releases too much dopamine at once. This means the receiving cell is unable to handle it. Overwhelmed, the receiving cell drops some of its receptors in self-defense, which reduces its ability to receive dopamine in the future.

You can think of it like a quarterback throwing a football to a receiver. In a healthy state, he'll catch it every time, but when on porn, it's like a quarterback throwing ten footballs simultaneously to the receiver. The receiver becomes so overwhelmed that he doesn't catch any of the footballs.

So in the future, when experiencing everyday simple pleasures like a hot meal, walking by an attractive woman, playing the guitar, reading a good book, talking socially, your brain isn't able to receive the dopamine stimulus that it once did, leading to a numbed experience feeling of life.

All in all, excessive porn use leads to less dopamine being able to travel through your brain, leading to desensitization. When this happens, dopamine has a harder time moving in your brain, regardless of the reason it was sent out. This desensitizes you not only to porn but everything in your life that would normally give you pleasure through a dopamine response. Excessive porn reduces dopamine flow, which reduces motivations and makes you feel less excited and satisfied when you do things you used to enjoy.

And with reduced pleasure and motivation from daily tasks, you feel apathetic, lethargic, and overwhelmed. Life appears to have lost its luster, and when it reaches a certain point, apathy turns into full-blown depression, with you becoming increasingly reliant on pornography to make you feel better, even if only for a short time.

Once you're in a state of depression, you begin to isolate yourself, live in a constant state of sadness, despair and feel overwhelmed, which creates an unhealthy environment. In this environment, it is extremely difficult to thrive in your personal and professional life.

Watching porn gives you a massive dopamine stimulation that you typically won't get from anything else in your day-to-day life. Work is so-so tiring, going to the gym gives you a temporary boost, but it's a lot of work; watching television is boring, so porn has become the only outlet that seems to give you pleasure. Not to mention it becomes the most exciting part of your day and, for many, a daily ritual.

Nothing you do during your day will come nearly as close to the dopamine rush you get from porn, so things you once found stimulating are increasingly boring. Learning to play the guitar is stressful... Learning that second language is mundane... Going to the gym is tedious... Learning to salsa dance seems tiresome... Improving your professional network is trite... Going to that local comedy club seems uninteresting...

Things that used to bring joy to your life simply have less importance to you as you consume more and more porn. And the problem here is the more porn you consume, the more desensitized to life you become.

Throughout your day, you're constantly looking forward to getting home and watching porn. You might leave work excited that you get to go home and watch porn, you might be leaving a social venue with friends excited to go home and watch porn, you might be on a date excited to go home and watch porn. You might even be having sex thinking about porn to get you off. What's happening here is you are looking forward to porn rather than looking forward to life.

Porn has caused such an imbalance in your life that once everyday pleasures are now seen as mundane, boring, and pointless. Porn has become the shiny object of desire that you look forward to rather than your personal goals or ambitions. You still even may be pursuing goals in your life, but they feel forced and unnatural.

Porn just feels right, so it's this constant urge to consume more porn. You do it, but then soon after you're bored, so you do it again and again. This spiral of negative actions leads you to feel more guilt and shame about how you've spent the last few hours watching porn. That lust for life is gone.

Imagine how you look to women after you've just watched two hours of porn, and now you're trying to go talk to that beautiful woman in her pretty dress. No wonder she didn't give you the time of day...

A porn addict is not living in the real world; he's living for that next scene. The good news is that stopping or significantly reducing porn and masturbation use and living a healthy, well-balanced lifestyle can restore your brain to its normal function. When you stop the porn, the receptors grow back, and your brain can resensitize itself to dopamine again with time. It can take months, but it can still happen, and you can live happily again.

Porn cannot only desensitize you to life, but it also causes problems sexually with women. Here's how...

THE TRUTH

Porn has been known to cause these problems in men: avoiding or lacking interest in sex with a real partner, experiencing difficulty becoming sexually aroused with a real partner and maintaining erections, or even unwanted delayed orgasm.

Men can feel the need to think of porn during sex to

get off or be too aggressive, demanding, or rough with a partner trying to act out porn fantasy. Men can become emotionally distant and not present during sex, feeling dissatisfied following sex with a real partner, which leads to having difficulty establishing or maintaining an intimate relationship. Overall, porn can desensitize you to sex with a woman since real sex may not be as exciting as porn, and you've trained your brain to be stimulated by porn and masturbation, not real sex.

Porn is also unrealistic. Women in porn do things that not all women in the real world want to do. Not every woman wants to be a man's sex slave every time, to give blowjobs on command, or to ejaculate on their face or have a penis in their ass. These are, of course, normal acts in porn, and you have trained your brain to expect and want these things from women. Regular sex for many becomes boring and less stimulating than watching porn and masturbating.

Watching excessive amounts of porn has led to men having erectile dysfunction and prolonged ability or inability to ejaculate with real women. Your brain needs dopamine to have and maintain an erection, and if you have become desensitized from porn, then your brain is not receiving the dopamine it needs to have and maintain an erection. Equally, your brain also needs dopamine to ejaculate. If your brain is desensitized, then this can lead to prolonged ejaculation.

Frequent and compulsive masturbation can also desensitize a man to common types of touch and stroke. When this happens, normal vaginal stimulation doesn't work, and it becomes difficult to maintain sexual stamina and interest. If a man continues down the path of watching more and more porn and masturbating, then a real vagina no longer pleasures as good as the grip of your hand and the visual stimulation of the unending novelty of porn.

When a healthy male has sex, arousal builds up through different triggers that respond to sight, sound, and touch. As the sex intensifies, the arousal builds until it reaches the point of ejaculatory ecstasy. If porn use has desensitized your brain to dopamine, then arousal won't build up enough for you to ejaculate. You can also be so harsh on your penis when you masturbate that you have become less sensitive to stimulation through touch. You shouldn't have erectile dysfunction if you're under the age of 40 and in good health. If you can only get an erection to porn, then porn could be the main source of this problem.

Don't mask the problem by investing in erection supplements and drugs. Solve the problem at its roots by significantly reducing or stopping porn and masturbation use.

Your body can recover itself from the damage caused by porn over the course of months or years. Begin that journey and start to experience harder and longer-lasting erections and enjoy ejaculation with women in the real world versus porn.

Porn doesn't just reduce your ability to perform in the bedroom but also damages your views of women. If you've struggled in dating or in relationships with women, then the next chapter could be the root of the problem.

12

LOOKING AT WOMEN LIKE SEX OBJECTS INSTEAD OF HUMANS

Objectification is a critical reason why an abuser tends to get worse over time.

— LUNDY BANCROFT

The more porn we watch, the more of an obsession we develop, looking at women as objects to be fucked rather than interacting with women as the beautiful, intellectual, unique individuals they are.

Dr James B. Weaver stated before the U.S. "Prolonged exposure to pornography in men creates and enhances sexual callousness toward women," wrote the Senate in 2004. Porn leads to a loss of respect for female sexual autonomy as well as men's lack of inhibition in expressing aggression toward women."

Women are soon objectified and rated solely by size, shape, and hip-to-weight ratio, which destroys any type of emotional availability and real connection with a woman.

Men feel this strong need to validate their masculinity

by how physically beautiful their woman is regardless of her values. This gives the idea that women are trophies or collectibles to show the world who a man is. And by watching porn, they only reinforce the idea that women's bodies are trophies and objects.

Women become objectified when you look at women as sex objects and view marriage or being in an official relationship as a license for unlimited sex. Every woman becomes a fantasy in your head, sometimes instantly. You can always tell when a man is addicted to porn simply by how he looks at a woman. He talks at her instead of with her, and he stares at her physical features. The way he tries to get something from her instead of building something with her.

Frequent porn use brings about the fear of deep intimacy with women and even social friendships. Men have developed an inability to relate with women in an honest, authentic, and intimate way despite being very lonely and yearning for this level of deeper connection inside. All in all, this happens because porn overpowers a man's needs over deeply intimate connections in their relationships.

Have you ever heard a woman say, "You're emotionally unavailable," or she checked out of the relationship even though you met all of her needs on paper (house, car, good job, friends, family)? This is exactly what this means. Bottom line: If you want to have a deep, long-lasting connection with a woman, you have to stop and significantly reduce your porn use and masturbation.

Additionally, men who watch porn like to isolate themselves as they prefer a plethora of virtual women over interacting with a real woman. It's easier and less stressful in the short term. Escaping the responsibilities of being a normal human being with friends and women is exactly what it means to lose your soul. You're losing your humanity, actually.

Boys grow up inundated with messages from porn that objectify women's bodies and depict women as sex objects who solely exist for male stimulation and pleasure. For many men, they don't understand that what they're doing is wrong since they've been programmed this way for decades by porn and mainstream media's acceptance of sex culture.

If you respond to sexual triggers by turning to porn, then you've taught your brain to expect overstimulation whenever those triggers happen. Any sexual trigger now causes a much stronger reaction than the trigger should call for.

The more porn you watch, the more triggers it places in your mind until everything reminds you of sex. When you see high heels, lipstick, a skirt, a cheerleader outfit, or a girl bending over to tie her shoe, you think about porn, sending you down a spiral of fantasy and horniness tempting you to watch more porn.

Depression and dopamine desensitization affect the part of your brain responsible for selecting what to pay attention to. When only porn and things related to porn can muster a strong dopamine response, triggers unrelated to pornography are considered less important.

If you spend one hour per day watching porn, you may interact with women more virtually than in real life, making it more difficult for you to connect with women.

For instance, when you're looking at women, you

concentrate and stare at her breasts, lips, and buttocks. You anticipate her to take her clothes off, you fantasize about her moaning and pay no attention to what's going on, and you're not present at all – you're in your head playing a sexual fantasy. And she's looking at you like, "what the f*ck is this guy doing?"

What's more, men believe they should make love like a pornstar. Porn is a performance, an act, not an emotional, intimate connection to cherish. Porn gives you what you want and makes you want things you never thought you'd want before.

And when you do interact with a woman, it's in a sexual way, or at least you want it to be in a sexual way. This can leave you powerless where sexual impulses control your life, fantasies pop up all of the time, and there's nothing you can do other than let them play out and try to act normally and respectfully.

This changes how you communicate with women in the real world and often in a negative way that doesn't serve what you truly want: a fulfilling and loving relationship with a woman. For example, when a woman tells you about her day, you're fantasizing about turning her around and throwing her up against the wall, hearing her scream your name, and cumming on her face.

The woman might not know that you're having hyper-sexual thoughts, but she senses something's not right. This sensation can make her feel uncomfortable just being around you, preventing you from becoming a friend, professional contact, or even romantic partner.

All in all, porn decreases the quality of your relationships with women in the real world. To achieve the same level of sexual arousal with a woman, you need your sex to become more extreme – more like porn. Partners of compulsive porn users often complain that their partners need increasingly risky, violent, and degrading sexual acts to get off. This puts your partner in a tough position: Do they accept this behavior in fear of losing you or stand up and also lose you?

This situation forces the woman to make choices she doesn't want to make. She feels second to your sexual desire and wonders if you are really into her or you just are using her as an outlet to gratify your sexual fantasies. She may wonder, is she your fuck toy or your lover?

When real sex with real partners becomes less interesting, it forces you to go back to porn because you can get what you want. And porn not only damages your views of women but equally has a negative effect on yourself as a man, and here's why...

THE MALE PORNSTAR'S ROLE IN ALL OF THIS

The male porn actor teaches you to be heartless, apathetic, amoral and entitled to use women in any way you want. He teaches you to demonstrate zero empathy, respect, or love for the women you have sex with, no matter how comfortable or in pain the woman is.

After sex, the male ejaculates and then leaves. There is no sign of intimacy with the women whose face he has ejaculated on. Porn does a good job of reducing the male and only focusing on the female to make it feel like the viewer is the male in the movie. This accentuates the male gaze, like a first-person perspective.

This leads men to try to be that guy in the porn film when they are having sex with a woman. The problem is the average man does not have a fully erect hard 10" penis that can last for 45 minutes. Male pornstars are typically on Viagra or Caverject, a type of direct penis enhancement injection, and other supplements to keep their penis fully erect and prolong ejaculation (please don't get any ideas now).

The average sex in normal life lasts 10 minutes, so don't be too tough on yourself if you're not King Kong lasting for hours. By watching a man with a large penis lasting long and the women screaming and enjoying (really acting) the sex, a lot of men have trained themselves to believe that this is how you sexually please women.

The problem here is that this isn't what really works and what all women want from sex. Many women prefer the average length of an erect penis of 4 to 6 inches. In fact, 90% of all men in the world have a penis between 4 to 6 inches.

Anything smaller or bigger makes up the other 10%. And not every woman wants to have sex for an hour and would prefer only 10 to 15 minutes because sex longer than that can often be painful.

All in all, you don't need to be tough on yourself if you ejaculate after 5 to 10 minutes and if your penis is average in size. Sex is not only about penetrating a woman, but also the touch, skin, breathing, talking, hair, being naked and vulnerable, all in the heat of the moment.

Also, when a man watches porn, it makes him feel like a beta male, a spectator who gets rewarded for something he didn't earn. You are watching another man having sex, and this is getting you off. Instead of watching other men have sex, you need to become the type of man who is having the type of healthy sex life he wants.

This is like watching those shows that show rich people's houses, cars, and boats. Don't watch that stuff in envy of those people. Instead, start taking action and becoming the type of man who deserves those things (if that is what you want).

"A man who wastes one hour of his life has not discovered the meaning of life," says Charles Darwin. The more porn you watch, the more you're training yourself to be a beta male.

Porn has filled a man's daily existence with more and more distractions. Instead of taking action towards their goals, men find that porn takes them farther and farther from the core of the man they want to be.

To sum it up, be a courageous action taker in your life versus a spectator who will be in the same place 5 or 10 years from now. Not only does watching porn make you feel like a beta male, but it can also ruin a core pillar of your health, causing you to lose the energy you need so you can work hard on your goals the next day.

13

WHY PORN GIVES YOU THE
WORST SLEEP EVER

A ccording to Pornhub.com, the largest tube porn site in the world, between the hours of 10 p.m. and 12 a.m., there is a surge in pornographic activity, which is generally the hours most people go to sleep. The problem is when dopamine increases at night, it delays melatonin production in your body. Melatonin is the hormone that regulates your sleep and wake cycles.

Melatonin production kicks in around 10 p.m. for most people, so if you are watching porn and masturbating, then you are releasing dopamine, which gets you excited, alert, and awake instead of preparing for sleep. So although you may feel relaxed and fall asleep after climaxing to porn, it's a restless type of sleep.

This means that your body will start producing melatonin later in the night, so when you wake up in the morning at 7 a.m., your body still has melatonin inside. This means you wake up feeling groggy, in brain fog, and lethargic. And it's not because you didn't sleep enough hours but because you did not get restful sleep.

And since your body still has melatonin inside, it might not fully go away until 10 a.m. to noon, so you've spent your entire morning in a hazy rut, and you don't fully wake up until the middle of the day.

In this situation, you've spent half of your day in a "slump," and you might be thinking that you're feeling depressed or you've got some problems. But really, it's because you got restless sleep due to watching porn late at night. If you were to abstain from watching porn late at night, then you would notice an increase in energy and alertness in the mornings.

HOW PORN PREYS ON YOU

The big question I often get is why do men still watch porn despite knowing the consequences?

For some, knowing is not enough, and there is something deeper going on in his life, so a man may continue watching porn to fill an emotional void in his life.

This is often attributed to a lack of intimacy with a partner, family, or friends. Men who are emotionally unavailable typically will be more vulnerable to watching porn and becoming addicted.

Like any addiction, porn can easily prey on a man who needs a quick hit of instant gratification or some dopamine to feel excited about life for a short while. People are very vulnerable to becoming porn addicts if they meet any of the following: prior addictive behavior in family to drugs, alcohol, food or gambling, history of neglect, history of emotional, physical, or sexual abuse, social anxiety, depression, attention deficit disorder, obsessive-compulsive disorder, or history of self-harm behaviors.

Also, men who live out of alignment with what they should be doing with their lives or who live off-purpose (basically wasting time or doing something they shouldn't be doing with their lives like a bad job or involved in a toxic relationship) are vulnerable to porn addiction.

It can be very easy to just click over on a new tab and start watching porn. It's fun, gratifying, and of course, it's too easy to acquire that dopamine hit to make you feel good at the moment. The key here is to acknowledge what challenges you have and start working on them to improve your life.

Typically heavy porn users watch porn because they are trying to mask some other serious life challenge. While there is no easy remedy for all of the above life struggles, you can recognize your failures and begin working on them right away. Then in time, you will overcome any challenge.

For however long you live in an unhealthy state, you will always be very susceptible to watching porn. If you improve your life, then you can decrease your desire to watch porn – your life, not porn, becomes your stimulus for dopamine.

You might have heard of the term "addicted2life," and hey, that's not a bad thing to love the life you've created for yourself. Note that not all depression and social challenges are caused by porn, but it can add to your depression, and it certainly doesn't help the problem. It's like pouring fuel over a fire – it's only going to magnify the problem.

And you may have been told you have a problem or special medical condition going on, but it could be really driven by your addiction to porn.

14

THE PATH TO RECOVERY

By now, I'm sure you understand the overall effects of sexual addiction, porn, and masturbation, and you're ready to make some changes to improve your life. If you have been watching porn for more than one year – which is probably the case with 99% of men reading this book – then it's going to be difficult to just quit cold turkey. You may be able to do this for two weeks or a month, but your cravings and withdrawals will be so hard that it would be easy for you to watch porn again.

And you may try it again, and then the same thing will happen. You may get to a point where you give up and declare that you're going to watch porn for the rest of your life.

I recommend a long-term, sustainable plan to let go of porn and masturbation with three main focus areas:

- Limit the amount of time you spend watching porn.
- Reduce the time spent watching porn.

• Reduce the number of scenes you watch.

Also, stop fast-forwarding or skipping to the parts you want to watch. Anticipation is healthier for you than the instant stimulus of going straight into penetration and ejaculation. You need to eliminate that novelty factor of porn, which fuels your addiction. The goal is to make watching porn unenjoyable and less novel and to spend less time doing it.

Never again allow yourself to go on a porn binge for hours. Make a declaration to yourself right now that the porn binges are a thing of the past, and you are now going to commit to cutting back on porn use and masturbation. I want you to push yourself to get back into the real world to replace pornographic stimulus with real-world stimulus to rewire your brain back to a healthy functioning state.

Here's how to do this:

Stage 1: Cut the number of times you watch porn, the time spent, and the number of scenes in half.

For example, a heavy user may watch porn four times per day, 30 minutes each time, and watch ten scenes each time. So cut it in half to 2 times per day, 15 minutes each session, and only five scenes.

Stage 2: Once per day for 8 minutes and only three scenes for 30 days.

Stage 3: Every other day for 8 minutes and only two scenes for 30 days.

Stage 4: Once per week for 8 minutes and only two scenes for 30 days.

Stage 5: Every other week or twice per month for 8 minutes and only 1 scene for 30 days.

Stage 6: Once per month for 5 minutes and only 1 scene for 90 days.

For many, Stage 5 is a healthy place to be – you are only watching porn every other week (twice per month). This would be considered a huge win for any former porn addict.

If you find yourself falling short, then simply reset your 30 days. It's okay if you're stuck at any stage for 60 or even 90 days. Ideally, you can get to stage 6 in about nine months, but if it takes you 12 months or longer, then there is nothing wrong with that either.

Everyone has their journey, but the key is that you started, and you have to remember being at Stage 4 is much better than where you were last year. Don't be too hard on yourself – just don't give up or think this isn't something you can't do.

I believe the only way someone will quit watching porn and masturbating forever is when they create a life of their choosing and live their best life. When a man receives his stimulus from healthy sex life, has strong friendships, loves his work, and is financially free (not a millionaire but just doesn't worry about money), and pursues his passions, there is little room for porn and masturbation.

My ultimate goal for you is not only to stop watching porn and masturbating but to use this extra free time to focus on creating the life of your dreams. Whatever that looks like, go in that direction and become the best man you can be.

❧ 15 ❧

LONG TERM HEALING FROM
SEXUAL ADDICTION

For most sex addicts in the process of healing, sexual recovery has distinct stages that are moved through in fits and starts. For instance, in the first few weeks and months of healing, sex addicts are typically focused on the basic steps of separating themselves from both their denial and problematic behaviors, defining what sexual sobriety means for them, developing and implementing a personalized sexual boundary plan, and finding useful therapeutic assistance. As recovery progresses and sex addicts become more comfortable living within the bounds of their personalized plan for sexual recovery, things like friendships and romantic relationships become more important.

As discussed throughout this book, sexual addiction, at its core, is little more than a maladaptive attempt to simply feel okay in an individual who struggles with shame, self-esteem, intimacy, and emotional self-regulation.

When viewed this way, it is easy to understand that long-term recovery must address these issues in meaningful ways. In other words, the keys to lasting sexual sobriety lie beyond the formation of a sexual boundary plan. Long-term healing is a lot about creating and deepening the kinds of relationships required for long-term accountability. As such, sex addicts who truly desire long-term sexual sobriety and a better life will agree to be fully honest with and take advice from other people.

Sometimes they may be asked to implement constraints that irk them, that they may not see a need for, and becoming accountable for their actions to people they barely even know, all because they truly wish to heal from their addiction.

The good news is that even those who are only going through the motions of sexual sobriety to please others—spouses, employers, legal officials, and so on—can profit from the early stages of recovery.

Even if they continue to act out in secret, as many of these individuals choose to do, they still, at the very least, become aware that active sexual addiction becomes harder and harder to conceal and that living a double life grows ever more stressful. They also tend to see that over time compulsive sexual behavior becomes less and less enjoyable and less effective as a means of emotional self-soothing.

In Alcoholics Anonymous, they sometimes say that nothing is worse than a belly full of booze and a head full of recovery. This is also true with sexual addiction. Once the addict knows that he or she has a problem, compulsive sexual behaviors lose their appeal. As soon as the addict's denial begins to crack, sexually addictive behaviors can never again occur without at least a tiny understanding that "this is a very bad idea and I really need to stop."

Eventually, of course, sex addicts must fully commit to a recovery process (like it or not), or they will continue sliding into the ever-deepening downward spiral of their addiction. Those who opt for the former nearly always find that their lives steadily get better by taking steady steps forward. And those who opt for the latter nearly always experience a continuing and ever-escalating series of negative life consequences. If they are lucky, they may eventually return to the recovery and healing process with a true commitment to change.

UNDERSTANDING SLIPS AND RELAPSE

Sadly, slips and relapses are common, almost expected, in early recovery from sexual addiction. As such, it is important for sex addicts (and their loved ones) in the process of healing to understand that temporarily backsliding into the psychological pull of addiction is not the end of the world, nor does it implies that they have failed.

Instead, it's an opportunity for them to learn and reaffirm, if not reinforce, their determination to live differently in the future. Yes, some sex addicts are lucky. They create their boundary plans and stick to them right from the start. However, most experience at least a few bumps in the road, slipping or relapsing at least once or twice. Something no spouse ever wants to hear or accept, but it is important to acknowledge and accept that the addict remains honest about their struggles. Either way, the process of recovery and healing is about progress rather than perfection. No addict ever recovers perfectly, nor should any sex addict ever expect to do so. Note that this statement *is* not an excuse to slip.

Sex addicts should also be aware that slips and relapses are not the same thing. Let's take a look at the differences here:

SLIP:

This is an unintentional, brief return to addiction. A slip may occur due to an unwanted stressor or a poorly designed sexual-boundary strategy that leads toward rather than away from triggers. An immediate and truthful disclosure will help handle and contain a slip.

After a slip, recovering sex addicts must tell others—therapists, twelve-step sponsors, accountability partners, spouses, and supportive friends in recovery (including their spouses!)—about the event if they hope to get back on track. Like it or not, honesty is absolutely key here to prevent the progression of the disorder!

RELAPSE:

By definition, a relapse is a series of slips that occur one after another, most often because an addict keeps that first one secret, choosing to minimize, rationalize, hide and justify his or her behavior over integrity and honesty. Their secrets and concealment set the stage for a wide variety of relapse patterns to manifest with increasing frequency and severity. The addict is soon back where he or she began: dealing with full-fledged, out-of-control sexual addiction.

Common warning signs for slips and relapse include:

- **Overconfidence:** "This is going really well. Maybe I have the problem licked."
- **Denial:** "See, I can stop my sexual acting out without any trouble. Now that I've proved this, I can look at porn like a normal person without worrying about consequences."
- **Isolation:** "I'm capable of doing this on my own." I don't need to attend counseling or 12-step sessions, and I don't need to be in close touch with other sex addicts in recovery."
- **Blaming:** "I wouldn't feel the need to go online to socialize if my spouse hadn't gotten the new work that takes up too much of his/her time and energy."
- **Making Excuses:** "I realize that being alone with my computer is a dangerous situation, but I need to remain late at work to finish this important project."
- **Setting Up Slippery Situations:** "The buffet at that Chinese restaurant across the street from where the prostitutes hang out is really good, so I'm going to have lunch there alone today."
- **Minimizing:** "I'm only looking at a little porn. It's not like I've gone back to having affairs with real people."
- **Ignoring or Devaluing Feedback from Supportive Others:** "The people in my counseling and 12-step groups are just interested

in controlling me. The things they want me to do might work for them, but they have no idea who I am or what I'm going through."

- Victimized: "I don't understand why I have to deprive myself when everyone else can watch porn and have webcam sex without fear of being judged."

- **Rationalizing:** "It's okay for me to 'step out' when I'm traveling for work or on vacation. My' rules for sobriety' don't count when I'm in a different state, and besides, no one will know."

- **Ignoring Previously Agreed-Upon Guidelines:** "I know I told my wife I wouldn't watch porn or flirt with other women on hook-up apps, but she can't hurt herself if she doesn't know."

- **Feeling Entitled:** "I've been working really hard on my recovery for six months, and I've been working double shifts at work, and no one seems to notice the effort I'm putting forth." I've earned a little treat for myself."

As mentioned above, slips and relapse are not the end of the world, though they often feel like failures and feel shameful to discuss. Rather than seeing these incidents as unsolvable disasters, recovering sex addicts (and their support networks) should see them as the opportunities for progress that they are.

To put it another way, setbacks should be regarded as issues to be explored and resolved rather than personal shortcomings. As a consequence, after a slip or relapse, addicts will (step by step) explore the "stinking thinking" that led to their relapse, recognize the trigger or triggers that pushed them over the edge, and devise ways to treat themselves better in the future if the same or a similar situation occurs, with the help of knowledgeable others. They should also consider other scenarios in which they could relapse and devise strategies for dealing with them. They should tighten their sexual boundary strategy if appropriate.

Whatever the case may be, any recovering addict who experiences a fall or relapse should immediately get honest with his or her therapist, family, twelve-step sponsor, and social support group about what's going on. Recovering sex addicts establish these loving and empathetic connections for a reason; now is the time to use them. If a sex addict in the midst of a slip or relapse is unable or unwilling to ask for help and fully own up to their challenges, his or her downward slide will almost certainly continue. If, however, that person reaches out and asks for assistance, he or she can save his or her sexual sobriety, along with the good life that accompanies it.

BASIC TOOLS OF SEXUAL RECOVERY: COPING MECHANISMS

Unfortunately for sex addicts, sexual triggers are unavoidable, as sex is so thoroughly baked into our consumer culture. In today's world, anyone, anywhere, anytime can be triggered into sexual desire: driving past one sexy billboard after another, seeing someone showing just a bit too much skin at the mall, sitting in the stands at a kid's soccer match, picking up a magazine at a friend's house, hanging out at a neighborhood party, attending a work event, taking the dog for a walk, going to the movies, working out, sitting at home watching TV, picking up a cell phone, driving through a particular neighborhood, etc. Triggers are endless in number and variety, and there is quite literally nothing to be done about this beyond learning what it feels like to be triggered and how to implement healthier (i.e., non-addictive) coping choices when needed.

When sex addicts are triggered, it is important that they have a "recovery toolbox" that they can reach into in their moment of crisis. After all, utilizing one or more healthy coping mechanisms (tools of recovery) is the only consistently effective way to short-circuit the addictive cycle. A few essential tools for recovering sex addicts include (but are not even remotely limited to) the following:

- Utilizing a Recovery or Accountability Partner: Addiction is best chased into remission by honesty, vulnerability, and transparency with another person who is aware of the problem and utilized as a sounding board, support person, co-decision-maker (around sexual and romantic choices), etc. To go it alone most often means remaining addicted or trading one addiction for another. It takes practice and hard work to consistently reach out to another person for direction, especially when related to sexual decision-making (private, personal, etc.). But it must be done and with the right person, someone who is non-shaming but unafraid to give unfiltered, honest feedback. Addicts are far too good at convincing themselves that things are "okay," whereas a neutral, caring outsider would clearly not see them as "okay." Therapists, sponsors, long-term friends, and clergy often can serve in this role. As stated, it is best not to give this task to a spouse or romantic partner, as they are too personally involved to be neutral and nonjudgmental when giving direction and advice.

- The Sexual Boundary Plan: Sexual boundary plans are created for several reasons—helping addicts to understand the nature of their addiction and to define their personal version of sexual sobriety, identifying "slippery" areas to watch out for, and providing addicts with guidance when they are triggered and unsure of what to do next. Many sex addicts carry printed or digitized versions of their boundary plan with them at all times. That way, if/when addicts feel triggered, they can look at their inner boundary and see that a particular behavior is prohibited. More importantly, they can look at the outer boundary and find a handy list of alternative activities. For most sex addicts, even a quick glance at certain outer boundary items—"re-earn the respect and trust of my wife and kids," for instance—is enough to halt the addictive cycle.
- Twelve-Step Sexual Recovery Meetings: To

maintain long-term recovery, sex addicts need places where they can talk openly and honestly, without fear of judgment, about their addiction, including when, where, why, and how they are sometimes triggered. This is doubly true after they've been triggered and then struggled to halt the addictive cycle. By far, the most readily available safe (empathetic, nonjudgmental, and relatively private) place to do this is before, during, or after group therapy or a twelve-step sexual recovery meeting. Put simply, one of the most powerful tools in the box is talking to another recovering sex addict. And if no meeting is taking place at that moment, addicts can turn to their group's phone list and call anyone on it. Having this handy list of phone numbers of supportive friends in recovery is essential when addicts have an urge to act out, when they need immediate help in a crisis, or when they simply want support and guidance from someone who "speaks their language."

- HALT: This means Hungry, Angry, Lonely, and Tired. Any of these simple conditions can leave an addict more vulnerable than usual to acting out. Let's face it: when hunger, frustration, loneliness, or fatigue clouds their judgment, even healthy, non-addicted people tend to act in ways they might later regret. The trick here is for addicts to recognize and address these needs when they arise, rather than simply lumping them in with every other form of emotional discomfort that they don't want to experience (and once tried to avoid by acting out sexually). As such, especially when triggered in early recovery, sex addicts must learn to HALT and ask themselves: When was the last time I ate something? Is it true that I didn't get enough sleep the night before? Is there a problem that needs to be resolved in my life? Can a few minutes of chatting with someone who knows what I'm going through make me feel better? A catnap, a candy bar, or a five-minute phone call can almost always dramatically reduce the desire to act out sexually.

- Self-Care: It can be difficult to think of someone who is having a great deal of sex as being "deprived." But it is a fact that most active addicts of all stripes can and will ignore even their most basic physical needs (eating, sleeping, daily showers, etc.) in order to remain engaged in their addiction of choice. Thus a defined routine of self-care that is inclusive of diet, exercise, medical check-ups, recreation, and fun (alone and with others) are as important to keeping an addiction in check as are all the don'ts and don'ts and can'ts that are in place to discourage problem behavior.

- "Bookending" Difficult Events: Sometimes sex addicts are triggered unexpectedly. Other times, triggers can be anticipated long in advance. For instance, attending a social engagement where people will be looking their best and drinking alcohol is an obvious potential trigger for most sex addicts. Knowing this, addicts can arrange to "bookend" such an event with phone calls to their therapist, twelve-step sponsor, accountability partner, and another supportive person in recovery. An alcoholic commits to sobriety during the "before" call, and he or she may also make arrangements to prevent relapse in this specific situation. The "follow-up" call allows the addict to talk about what happened, how he or she felt, and what they can do differently next time. (Practicing bookending also helps with HALT's "lonely" portion.)

- Practicing Gratitude: Sex addicts have typically used their sexual fantasies and behaviors to numb themselves for so long that they've forgotten how to experience emotions—especially uncomfortable ones like anxiety, depression, shame, fear, and the like—in a healthy way. Sometimes, especially early in the recovery process, sex addicts can become overwhelmed by those feelings and lose sight of what is going right in their lives. Making a gratitude list is a perfect way to overcome this. Writing a ten-item appreciation list almost always works to combat every trigger and bring the addictive cycle to a halt. For some sex addicts, every gratitude list begins the same way: "I am grateful to be sober at this moment." Gratitude has the added advantage of promoting happiness. People who are grateful for what they have tend to focus on their strengths rather than their weaknesses, and they are in general more hopeful, less stressed-out, less likely to wallow in shame and depression, and more likely to recover from an addiction.

THE THREE-SECOND RULE

Sex addicts (just like the rest of us) are not in control of the thoughts and ideas that pop into their minds at any given moment. However, what they can control is how they act when they unexpectedly encounter problematic thoughts, triggers, or ideas. For instance, after recognizing that there is an unexpectedly attractive or seductively dressed person on the street, they can train themselves to do the following, rather than allowing themselves to "get into" addiction thinking (try it, it works well).

1st Second

Take one second to acknowledge that this is an attractive person or situation that you find arousing and a turn-on (sexual attraction is a natural part of being human that must be acknowledged, not shamed or avoided).

2nd Second

Look away. Look down or away, take this second to appreciate the sky, your surroundings, anything other than the object of your desire. Let yourself be aware that you are struggling, that you would rather keep staring at that person or get something (sexual) going with them or someone else. Allow the feeling, but instead of acting on it, take the opposite action by choosing to look away.

3rd Second

While still looking away, imagine in your mind that person as someone's daughter, granddaughter, nephew, son, etc. See them (in your mind, not by looking at them a second time) as a genuine, spiritual, real person worthy of love, who doesn't deserve to be used sexually or romantically and then thrown away.

Then keep moving on. By allowing the feeling, choosing to turn away, and then de-objectifying the person, you get to stay in the world and feel okay about yourself, as a healthy person with healthy sexual desires, who does not act on them every time you feel them, and as someone who appreciates that people are people, not objects. The more addicts practice this simple exercise, the easier it becomes to "be" in the world with less temptation and more hope.

Obviously, the half-dozen tools listed above are hardly the full kit. Journaling, written twelve-step work, ongoing outreach to others in recovery, twelve-step sponsorship (both giving and receiving), reading recovery-related literature, changing old routines, developing healthy hobbies, prayer, meditation, and just simply "thinking it through" are some of the hundreds of other tools. that sex addicts can use to combat their addictive patterns.

THE RECOVERY FROM GUILT AND SHAME

Sadly, sex addicts often feel shame (about who they are) rather than guilt (about what they have done). Meaning they believe something inside themselves is the root of their problem as if they are fundamentally flawed in some way and thus doomed to a life of suffering, loneliness, and regrettable behaviors. In certain cases, sex addicts in recovery need a significant amount of time before they can even begin to comprehend that they are not fundamentally flawed, that their addiction and its detrimental effects is triggered by their maladaptive choices rather than their true selves. Time is also needed for them to gain insight and empathy into the pain they have caused others. The good news is that once recovering addicts recognize that they are good people who have behaved badly rather than bad people who are just doing what bad people do, their recovery begins to accelerate.

It's important to remember that guilt and shame are not the same thing, particularly when it comes to recovery and healing. In fact, when a sex addict experiences guilt (rather than shame) after violating his or her core values—especially when the behavior has harmed not only the addict but other people—it demonstrates that the addict has a moral compass. Even better, the supposedly negative emotion of guilt can be a catalyst for long-term behavior change and lasting sexual sobriety.

Essentially, the desire to not experience the emotional pain wrought by guilt healthfully encourages all of us to not repeat past mistakes while also helping us develop empathy for others and a desire to make amends to those who've been harmed.

Unfortunately, many sex addicts live with profound internalized feelings of shame and self-loathing that are tied more to their inherent sense of self than to any specific activities or behaviors. These individuals often feel like bad, unlovable people, and that their problematic sexual behavior simply serves as proof of this fact. As this happens, a condition known as a shame spiral or narcissistic withdrawal restricts sex addicts from seeing beyond their self-loathing, causing them to spiral further into depression and loneliness, all of which are serious barriers to recovery.

The prevalence of shame spirals among sex addicts is one of the (many) reasons that social support is such an important element of the healing process. Put simply, shame does not occur in a vacuum. Instead, it occurs between people, and it, therefore, heals best between people. In fact, numerous studies have shown that discussing a traumatic/shaming event with a supportive person or people greatly reduces its short-and long-term negative effects. Dr John Briere, a long-time leader in trauma/shame research and treatment, has consistently stressed that it is not any specific traumatic event that causes the most stress and damage; it's how that event is handled within the family/community.

Dr Briere and many other clinicians have found that when traumatized and shamed, people share their most difficult experiences—the events that leave them feeling defective, unworthy, and unlovable—even long after the fact, their stress levels decrease, and their overall mental and physical health improves.

Of course, sharing about traumatic events and deep shame is, by nature, incredibly painful. As such, most people would "rather eat dirt" than talk about this stuff. Nevertheless, it is clear that shame, self-hatred, and self-loathing thrive in darkness but wither in sunlight. In other words, the best way to reduce the power of a shame-based self-image is to talk about shameful feelings and events with safe, supportive, empathetic others: the kinds of people that recovering sex addicts routinely encounter in sex-addiction-focused group therapy faith-based and twelve-step sexual recovery groups.

HOW TO GET BETTER

Like any addict who is mired in a problem of his own making, when a sex addict is ready to heal, he or she will nearly always require outside support and assistance. After all, if they could change their behaviors on their own (without help), they would do so, but they cannot. And this is not surprising when you understand the factors that drive the problem: primarily an unbroken cycle of triggers, acting out, and denial, plus a big dollop of lies, secrecy, shame, and self-loathing. To overcome these dynamics, addicts nearly always need the insight and the account-ability that only an objective outsider can provide. In short, shame and remorse about compulsive sexual behav-iors and even the worst related consequences are not enough to keep a sex addict from backsliding when chal-lenged by emotional and psychological discomfort.

Without external support, willpower alone just doesn't seem enough, and sex addicts' endless promises to change —made to themselves and others—almost inevitably fall by the wayside at some point.

The good news is that lasting behavior improvement and healthy life are entirely possible with the right advice and support. Before beginning this journey toward emotional healing and sexual recovery, it is important that sex addicts understand they will need to keep an open mind and become honest about their sexual thoughts and behaviors. This is never easy, of course, but it is always well worth the effort, as long-term healing from sexual addiction can foster a rediscovery of self and a much more rewarding creative, and connected life.

If sex addicts are married or in an otherwise committed relationship and a committed partner (despite their anger and hurt) is open to staying around and joining in the healing process, couple's recovery can help people appreciate emotional needs/desires, and that of their partner's more clearly while encouraging and allowing both parties to become more emotionally intimate with each other. Suppose sex addicts are not in a romantic relationship. In that case, recovery builds self-esteem and enables them to make healthier choices about dating, sexuality, and (if they so desire) the formation of a long-term intimate partnership.

As sex addicts heal from active addiction, honesty, integrity, self-knowledge, and a desire to be vulnerable and known for who they truly are, warts and all slowly but steadily replaces the double life they've been living. Secret lies and superficial connections fall away as they begin to feel better about their behavior and their self-identity. When taken on actively and honestly, sexual recovery can bring about unexpected levels of emotional maturity and hope for a future filled with loving, life-affirming friendships and romantic relationships. Admittedly, working toward change is not easy, especially when dealing with a deeply rooted addiction or a betrayed spouse, but it pays big dividends over time.

THE INITIAL STEP

Interestingly, even though sex addicts nearly always require outside assistance if they hope to heal, the first step on their healing journey is an internal one: deciding that they actually want help with their addiction.

Typically, this willingness to enter into the often difficult recovery process arises because the addict has experienced negative consequences related to his or her sexual behaviors. Often the addict's marriage or primary relationship, job, standing in the community, or freedom is threatened. Sometimes, motivation is internal, with the addict simply not liking the person they have become and wanting to change. It doesn't really matter where the initial impetus comes from—even superficial remorse (the desire to not get in any more trouble) can get the ball rolling—as long as there is a genuine motivation for change.

Once a sex addict is motivated to change and willing to accept outside assistance, it's time to get to work. This process starts with finding an accountability partner. An accountability partner is a person who holds the addict accountable for the work that must be done, often providing feedback as it happens. This supportive guide is typically a therapist, a twelve-step sexual recovery sponsor, a non-shaming clergy member, or a close friend who is also healing from sexual addiction. (For addicts not yet willing or ready to seek in-person assistance, certain websites and twelve-step groups offer online or phone support. But it is best to seek face-to-face help if/when available.) It is not advised for sex addicts to use a spouse or any other romantic partner as their accountability partner because those individuals are nearly always too close to the situation—and often too injured by the situation—to provide the objective input that is needed. This is true even when a spouse wishes to help.

Ultimately, the job of an accountability partner is to assist and guide the sex addict—in person, by phone, or even online—with identifying what his or her recovery-related commitments and priorities actually are and ways in which those commitments toward change can be met and maintained. Accountability partners are also there for support when sex addicts experience moments of weakness. As such, establishing and developing this connection is an essential element of growing and maintaining sexual recovery and healing.

A few of the more common and highly useful early-recovery commitments that an accountability partner might ask a sex addict to make include the following:

- Promise to reach out immediately if you feel triggered to act out sexually. (Feeling triggered is inevitable, and there is nothing wrong with it, so long as addicts start dealing with their triggers in a healthy, non-addictive way and not acting out their triggers.)
- Promise to reach out immediately if you actually do act out sexually. (Slips and relapse are common in early recovery from sexual addiction.) They must be honestly admitted and gleaned for insight.
- Throw away all physical material related to the

problem. (For instance, porn addicts need to throw out all books, magazines, VHS tapes, DVDs, flash drives, and other storage devices that contain pornographic imagery or stories, along with any related paraphernalia such as lubricants and sex toys. It is best to throw this material into a commercial Dumpster at least a mile from home. Sometimes accountability partners will supervise this process to ensure the addict does not enjoy the material one last time.)

- Go through your computer, laptop, tablet, smartphone, etc., deleting any and all files, emails, texts, sexts, bookmarks, profiles, apps, and contact information related to your addiction. Use the search capabilities built into your digital devices to look for these items. In other words, search for .gif, .tif, .jpeg, .wmv, .mpg, .mpeg, .mp4, .avi, and .mov files, among others. If possible, and if it won't disrupt other areas of your life, disable the webcams on these devices. (Again, accountability partners often supervise this process to make sure the addict does not "enjoy the material just one last time.")

- Cancel any sex addiction-related memberships to websites, apps, and brick-and-mortar establishments, along with any credit cards you've used to pay for these memberships to make sure they don't automatically renew. (If addicts don't want to cancel these cards, they can call the credit card company and report the card as lost. Credit card companies will gladly send replacement cards with different numbers, and this serves the same purpose as a cancellation.)

- Commit that you will stay away from "gray area" activities. (In the same way that alcoholics new to recovery should not hang out in bars, sex addicts shouldn't leave the Victoria's Secret catalog on the coffee table, frequent NC-17 movies, or get massages from strangers. People who are not sexually addicted can handle these things without becoming triggered; sex addicts cannot. So it is best to stay away from them.)

- Commit to only using digital devices where others can see you. At work and at home, orient computers and other digital devices so the screens are publicly visible. With portable digital devices, use them only in public places when others are around. (Recovering sex addicts need to understand that using these devices in private, even for a legitimate nonsexual purpose, is a gray area activity that could easily trigger the desire to act out.)

- Create reminders of why you want to change your behavior. Use pictures of your spouse or kids as background imagery on your digital devices. Use your wedding song or your spouse's voice as your ringtone, etc. (Visual and auditory reminders of what sex addicts stand to lose can be a powerful motivation for change.)

- Purchase and install "parental control

software." (These filtering, blocking, tracking, and accountability software products prevent access to problematic online venues and monitor a person's overall use of digital devices, typically providing reports to an accountability partner. See the Resources chapter for more information on these products.)

- Create and implement a plan for sexual sobriety. (This plan is best developed working in conjunction with the accountability partner. It'll almost certainly be in the form of a sexual boundary plan. Sexual boundary plans are discussed at length as this chapter progresses.)

SEXUAL SOBRIETY VERSUS SEXUAL ABSTINENCE

Sexual addicts in the early stages of recovery and healing typically have little to no idea what the term "sexual sobriety" actually means. Many worry that sexual sobriety mirrors chemical sobriety, where permanent abstinence from all mood-altering substances is required. In fact, sex addicts new to treatment often pose some form of the following question: "Will I still get to have a regular sex life?" or "Do I have to give up sex forever?" This question is usually followed by a statement like: "If I have to give up sex permanently, then you can forget about me staying in recovery." And who would fault them for this as sex is, after all, a natural life-affirming activity?

Fortunately, unlike sobriety for alcoholism and drug addiction, sexual sobriety is not defined by long-term abstinence. Instead, sexual addiction treatment addresses sobriety much as it is handled with eating disorders, another area in which long-term abstinence is simply not feasible. Essentially, instead of permanently abstaining from all sexual activity, recovering sex addicts learn to define and avoid being compulsive, problematic, objectified sexual behavior.

That said, sex addicts new to treatment and recovery are often asked to take a short timeout (usually thirty days or so) from all sexual behaviors, including masturbation, during which they begin the process of healing.

This brief period of total sexual abstinence is suggested because most have lost touch with reality when it comes to sexual behavior. Therefore, they can find it incredibly difficult to distinguish between healthy and problematic attractions, flirtations, and, of course, sex. This temporary celibacy period provides recovering sex addicts, working with a therapist or some other accountability partner, a chance to develop some clarity about which of their sexual behaviors are addictive and which are not. Sex addicts can also use this time to dismantle denial, learn what their triggers are, and develop healthy coping skills that they can turn to instead of acting out.

In much the same way that drug detox is a first step toward recovery from substance addiction, this short period of complete sexual abstinence—a "detox" from addictive sex—is a first step toward recovery from sexual addiction. This time away from sex (along with flirting, porn, cruising, emotional affairs, etc.) interrupts long-established patterns of compulsive sexual behavior while clarity, ego strength, social skills, support networks, and new coping skills are developed. Again, celibacy is not a long-term goal. In truth, the heavy lifting of sex addiction recovery is not this period of self-restraint; but rather, it's the slow (re)introduction of healthy sexuality and intimacy into the addict's life that takes the most work. In other words, the true goal of sexual recovery and sexual sobriety is not sexual celibacy; it's learning to meet one's emotional and physical needs without having to run to problematic sexual behavior as a quick fix for deeper issues.

CREATING A PERSONALIZED VERSION OF SEXUAL SOBRIETY

Many sex addicts new to the healing process openly wonder: "If sexual sobriety doesn't require priest-like celibacy, what does it require?" Interestingly, there is no cut-and-dried answer to this question. Each sex addict arrives in recovery with a unique life history and set of problems, along with highly individualized goals for his or her future life. Thus, each sex addict, with the help of his or her therapist or some other accountability partner, must craft a personalized version of sexual sobriety.

To create a personalized version of sexual sobriety, sex addicts must first delineate the sexual behaviors that do and do not compromise and destroy their values (fidelity, not hurting others, etc.), life circumstances (keeping a job, not getting arrested, etc.) and relationships. Sex addicts then undertake a written sexual sobriety contract pledging to indulge in only non-problematic sexual activities (for them). As long as their sexual behavior does not violate these highly individualized boundaries, they are sexually sober. It is important that these plans be put in writing and that they clearly define the addict's bottom-line problem behaviors. Murky plans lead to murky recovery, as does lack of accountability.

Once again, the definition of sexual sobriety, because it takes into account each person's values, beliefs, goals, and life circumstances, is different for every sex addict. For instance, sexual sobriety for twenty-eight-year-old single gay men will probably look very different than sexual sobriety for a forty-eight-year-old married father of three. The goal is not conformity; the goal is a non-compulsive, non-secretive, non-shaming sexual life.

DRAFTING THE SEXUAL BOUNDARY PLAN

Written sexual sobriety contracts often take the form of sexual boundary plans. These plans define and set limits on which sexual behaviors are and not acceptable for each individual sex addict. Typically, the process of crafting a sexual boundary plan begins with a statement of goals.

Essentially, sex addicts list the primary reasons they want to change their sexual behavior. A few commonly stated goals include:

- I want to spend my leisure time with my friends and family and have fun.
- I don't want to cheat on or keep secrets from my spouse.
- I want to be present in the real world and find a loving relationship instead of living my life online.

- I don't want to abuse pornography ever again.
- I no longer want to violate the rule (prostitutes, viewing illicit images).
- I want to feel like a whole, integrated, healthy person, living my life with integrity, not lies and manipulations.
- I don't want to worry about STDs anymore.

Once an addict's goals for recovery are clearly stated, he or she can move forward with the creation of a personalized sexual sobriety plan, utilizing these pre-established goals as an overall guide. Sometimes sexual sobriety plans are simple, straightforward statements like, "I will not engage in sexual infidelity no matter what," or, "I will not view pornography of any kind." More often, though, sex addicts require a more elaborate set of guidelines, typically a three-tiered plan, constructed as follows:

THE INNER BOUNDARY

This is the addict's bottom-line definition of sexual sobriety. Here a sex addict lists specific sexual behaviors (not thoughts or fantasies) that are causing problems in their lives and that they, therefore, need to stop. In other words, this boundary enumerates the harmful and troubling actions that have resulted in detrimental life outcomes and inexplicable demoralization for the addict. If the addict participates in inner boundary behaviors, their sobriety clock will need to be reset (while also doing a thorough examination of what led to the slip). A few common inner boundary behaviors are:

- Paying for sex
- Calling an ex for sex
- Going online for porn at work, home, or on my phone
- Engaging in webcam sex (paid or free)
- Getting sensual massages or hiring prostitutes
- Hooking up for casual or anonymous sex
- Having affairs
- Exhibiting oneself (online or real-world)
- Using apps to hook up with strangers

THE MIDDLE BOUNDARY

This boundary lists warning signs and slippery situations that might lead a sex addict back to inner boundary activities (acting out). Here the addict lists the people, places, thoughts/fantasies, events, and experiences that might trigger their desire to act out sexually. In addition to obvious potential triggers (logging on to the Internet when alone, driving through a neighborhood where prostitutes hang out, downloading a hook-up app, etc.), this list should include things that might indirectly trigger a desire to act out (working long hours, arguing with a spouse or boss, keeping secrets, worrying about finances, family holidays, etc.). A few common middle boundary items are:

- Skipping therapy and a support group meeting
- Lying (about anything), especially to a loved one
- Poor self-care (lack of sleep, eating poorly, forgoing exercise, etc.)

- Working more hours than usual or more intensely than usual
- Spending time with family of origin (holidays, reunions, etc.)
- Finding myself pushing those close to me away (irritability, fighting, creating unnecessary drama)
- Fighting or arguing with anyone, especially with loved ones
- Unstructured time alone
- Traveling alone (for any reason) without a plan to remain accountable
- Feeling lonely and unloved
- Feeling bored and restless

THE OUTER BOUNDARY

This boundary lists healthy behaviors and activities that can and hopefully will lead a sex addict toward his or her life goals, including things not at all limited to having a healthy, nondestructive sex life. These healthy pleasures are what the addict can turn to as a replacement for sexual acting out. Outer boundary activities may be immediate and concrete, such as "working on my house," or long-term and less tangible, such as "redefining my career goals." In all cases, the list should reflect a healthy combination of work community, recovery, and play. If going to a support group three or more times per week, exercising daily, and seeing a therapist one or more times per week are on the list, then spending time with friends, enjoying a hobby, and just plain relaxing should also be on the list. A few common (sample) outer boundary behaviors are:

- Spending more time with family, especially kids
- Reconnecting with old friends
- Rekindling an old hobby (or developing a new one)
- Getting in shape (exercise)—especially joining a team or group activity
- Getting regular sleep
- Working no more than eight hours per day
- Rejoining and becoming active in church/temple, *etc.*
- Going back to school
- Working on the house and yard—catching up on delayed plans
- Doing volunteer work

Every sex addict is different, and I cannot emphasize this enough. Each addict has his or her own life story, ambitions, and dysfunctional sexual habits. As a result, each sexual boundary plan is different. For one sex addict, profoundly disturbing behaviors may be perfectly appropriate for another and vice versa. As a result, there is no one-size-fits-all solution to sexual sobriety definition and practice. When developing a boundary plan, the key is for each addict to be fully, completely, and painfully honest with himself or herself.

It is important to also state that sexual boundary plans are about much more than staying away from inner boundary items (problem behaviors). Yes, eliminating problem behaviors is a primary and ongoing goal of recovery, but as the plan itself suggests, there is much more involved with the healing process than simply eliminating problem behaviors. That part should be considered a given. Over the long term, recovering from sexual addiction is much more about truly learning how to enjoy your life while healthfully coping with its daily ups and downs. After all, the outer boundary (above) defines how the addict wants to live his or her life. Put simply, no addict ever fully recovers simply by not doing certain things. The flip side is equally important. The more positive things a person does to feel good about themselves and life, the better their lives will be.

When first crafted, sexual boundary plans typically look airtight. However, they usually are not. And even when they are, many sex addicts find ways to manipulate and work around their plans. Knowing this, it is wise to keep the following tips in mind when constructing and implementing a sexual sobriety plan.

- **Be clear and specific.** Boundary plans are meant to define sexual sobriety and to set out a roadmap for living a healthy, happier life. They are contracts that are written and signed to keep sex addicts responsible to their commitments, particularly in the face of challenging circumstances. When sex addicts lack clearly written boundaries, they are vulnerable to decide at the moment that certain activities are okay for now, even though they've been wildly problematic in the past. Remember, impulsive sexual decisions made without clear guidelines are what dragged the addict down in the first place, so it's best not to leave any wiggle room in sobriety, especially in the first year.

- **Be flexible (over time).** Boundary plans are not set in stone. In reality, recovering sex addicts often spend a month (or a year) with a set of boundaries before realizing that their strategy needs to be modified. (Recent advancements in digital technology have prompted many long-term sex addicts to reconsider their plans.) However, changing a boundary plan is never something an addict can do on their own. The addict's therapist, twelve-step mentor, and accountability partner should always be consulted before making improvements. Changes to boundary plans are not made just because a "special situation" arises, and the addict wishes to make a change on the spur of the moment. This type of action is known as "acting out," not "changing the plan."

- **Be honest.** In order to develop good boundary strategies, not only the addict but also his or her advisors must be completely honest. Let's face it: if an addict wants to justify continuing a conduct even though he or she knows it doesn't serve a healthy purpose, he or she will almost always find someone to sign off on it (or at the very least accept that it's not a big deal). It's

important to remember that the goal
of creating a sexual boundary plan isn't to justify
and rationalize inappropriate behaviors (or even
watered-down versions of those behaviors) but
rather to put an end to sexual acting out and the
inexplicable demoralization that comes with it.

- **Consider others:** When a sex addict develops
their boundary plans while single, they often
find that they need to revise them once they
start a serious relationship. Sex addicts who
have been in long-term relationships should
think about how their new limits will affect
their partner. Explaining the reasons for these
apparently abrupt shifts in intimate relating
would normally help to mitigate the impact.

DO SEX ADDICTS EXPERIENCE WITHDRAWAL?

When alcoholics and drug addicts go "cold turkey," they
often experience withdrawal symptoms such as delirium
tremens (DTs), chills, fevers, insomnia, night sweats,
headaches, nausea, diarrhea, tachycardia (rapid heart rate),
hypertension, depression, agitation, anxiety, hallucina-
tions, irritability, and other symptoms. Withdrawal from
some drugs is more difficult than withdrawal from others.
The physical symptoms of opiate addiction (including
heroin addiction) and alcoholism are the most serious.
These symptoms may often be life-threatening if they are
not treated medically.

Substance users who are experiencing extreme physical
withdrawal symptoms are typically "titrated" off their drug

of choice, which means they are given a medication that "manages" their withdrawal by temporarily removing their addictive drug of choice and then gradually weaned off of it. This procedure will take anywhere from a few days to several weeks.

But what about sexual addiction. Do sex addicts get the DTs and hallucinate the same as alcoholics and heroin addicts? Typically they do not. This is not to say that abruptly ceasing to engage in addictive sexual fantasies and activities does not result in withdrawal. In truth, it almost always does, at least to some extent. Most often, withdrawal from sexual addiction manifests as one or more of the following:

- **Irritability, anxiety, agitation, depression, etc.:** Most sex addicts experience extreme emotional discomfort in early sobriety. And why not? After all, addictive sexuality has been their primary way of coping with any and all discomfort—including feelings as seemingly benign as boredom—for years on end. They no longer have this simple way of numbing out and escaping when the addiction is taken away. And if they don't have that, they'll have to confront their feelings head-on. For people who've been trying to "not feel" for years or even decades, this can be an incredibly uncomfortable experience both for them and those around them.
- **A desire to explore other potential addictions:** Many sex addicts new to recovery

find themselves replacing (or longing to replace) their sexual addiction with some other compulsive (and highly distracting) activity. Sometimes, this manifests as a cross-addiction. For instance, a sex addict who suddenly stops acting out experiences a corresponding flood of uncomfortable emotions (as discussed above), and he or she may turn to gambling, drinking, smoking, spending, drugging, eating, or any other pleasurable substance or activity if compulsive sexuality fails to stem the flow. Knowing this, it's critical for recovering sex addicts to keep a close eye on other pleasurable activities, especially during the first few months of recovery.

- **Loneliness and longing for connection:** For the majority of sex addicts, sexual acting out covers up not only everyday tension and emotional distress but also underlying problems such as a need for intimacy. This longer-term disorder can emerge without the continuous distraction of sexual fantasy and behavior, causing extreme feelings of loneliness, anxiety, isolation, and unhappiness. These emotions are entirely normal and expected. After all, sex addicts are grieving the loss of their primary long-term relationship (their addiction), and they naturally feel a need to replace it.

THE INITIAL STAGE ALWAYS TAKES WORK

In early sexual sobriety, even the smallest annoyance can feel like a major issue. Recovering sex addicts are likely to overreact and blow up if they don't have their go-to coping mechanism. They become enraged at themselves and others; they weep, become defensive, frightened, lonely, and so on. As such, sex addicts in early recovery are not always fun to be around. This is their emotional withdrawal.

In early recovery, some sex addicts, on the other hand, experience the polar opposite of withdrawal. This is referred to as the pink cloud or honeymoon. These fortunate individuals discover that once they begin the healing process, they lose all ability to act out sexually. They are fascinated by their insight into developing and thrilled to have finally found a solution to their deepest problem and someone to help.

This brief period of early recovery is fantastic while it lasts. Sex addicts riding the pink cloud, on the other hand, should be mindful that their urge to sexually act out will return, and it could be stronger than ever. It is possible to relapse or believe that something has gone wrong in the healing process if this eventuality is not expected and planned for. In fact, relapse is unnecessary, and recovery is perfectly fine. Instead, this is a natural part of the process, and the addict is actually going through a stage of withdrawal that is taking longer than usual.

Any sex addict who recognizes withdrawal symptoms should discuss them with a supportive person who is familiar with the sex addiction cycle. This person will often be a therapist, a twelve-step sponsor, or a friend in recovery.

It is often useful to be evaluated for depression or anxiety by a medical professional. Close friends and family members who are not in treatment can also be useful. If withdrawal symptoms are severe (especially depression, dissociation, and anxiety), seek help from a licensed mental health professional as soon as possible. Severe withdrawal symptoms left untreated can lead to relapse in sex addiction as well as other forms of severe self-harm.

16

FAIL PROOF RESOURCES TO
SUPPORT YOUR JOURNEY

Recovery is an ongoing process for both the addict and his or her family. In recovery, there is hope. And hope is a wonderful thing.

— DEAN DAUPHINAIS

1. Find a professional therapist trained in the treatment of addictions and sexual disorders. Sash.net is a place where you can find someone who can assist you one on one.
2. Find or create a support group in your community. Understanding that you are not alone on this journey is critical to overcoming this addiction. Note: You're not going through this alone – it's a very common challenge for everyone today.
3. Find an accountability partner where you check in with each other once per week. Share with him this book, and if he likes it, ask if he'd be interested in working on this together. There is no time here for the alpha male bravado "I can do this myself" mentality.

4. Throw out all physical material related to your problem. If you own any porn files, DVDs, external hard drives, sex toys, get rid of all of them. This might be hard to do for some, so what you can do is, at each new stage you enter, remove half of your entire collection every time.

5. With your accountability partner, each time you talk to each other, check in to see if they've done this and also if they've added anything new to their porn collection. If so, tell them to delete it immediately.

6. Cancel any membership to websites and apps. Save your money. I'd recommend spending it on healthier foods, a gym membership, a personal trainer, or a life coach.

7. Don't bring your smartphone or tablet into bed ever. If you have access to it, sometimes at night, when the lights are off, you can get these withdrawals and have a sudden and uncontrollable urge to do it at night. Keep all electronics in another room. This will also help you get better sleep.

8. Work in public more. Maybe after work, go to a trendy local coffee shop to surf the web instead of going home alone, which may trigger you to watch porn. I know it's more work, but if that's what it takes to make this happen for you, then it's worth it. Plus, it will make you more social anyways by getting out of your house and into the real world.

9. Around the house, display inspirational photos of family, fun events, and you having fun with friends. Give yourself a reason other than yourself why you're doing this. Sometimes we just need more, and that should give you constant reminders about who you love.

10. Whenever you have a sudden urge to watch porn, get

away from your computer or smartphone and stand up and take three deep breaths. Come back to the present moment and regain control of the urge. With each breath, notice the urge slowly fading away and channel this sexual energy into something productive.

11. Install filtering software and website blockers: Self-control for Mac, Getcoldturkey.com

12. Familiarize yourself with these online communities: sexualrecovery.com, assect.org, Reddit/nofap, reboot nation

If you have been using porn regularly, then withdrawal from porn can be filled with as much agitation, depression, and sleeplessness as detoxing from alcohol, cocaine, and other hard drugs. In fact, porn recovery can take up to 18 months, so take it one day at a time.

Notice your triggers. Someone recovering from AA shouldn't be found in a bar... a porn addict shouldn't be in an isolated dark room with a computer, tablet, or smartphone.

When you feel yourself wanting to watch porn, stop immediately what you are doing and admit you have entered a danger zone. If you are on your computer, then get up and away from the computer – get some fresh air, do some push-ups, and start doing something else right away, such as a small activity to end those thoughts.

Calm yourself physiologically and emotionally by taking five deep heavy breaths. And if you need to reach out for support, do it as quickly as possible. Always reaffirm your commitment to your recovery and that you will make it through the day. And celebrate the moments when you did pull away from a downward spiral and treat yourself to something you enjoy. This trains you to stop when you feel like you're about to watch porn.

Just admitting that you have a problem and want to improve makes you a man. This is taking responsibility for your life and pushing you closer to becoming the man you truly want to be.

17

RECOVERY RESOURCES, SUPPORT, AND EDUCATION

A
s mentioned repeatedly throughout this book, modern-day sexual addiction is a digitally driven endeavor. A decade or so ago, it was reasonable to suggest to sex addicts that they either stay away from computers altogether or use them only in very limited circumstances. But that was in the past, and this is in the present. In today's world, digital technology is an increasingly essential part of healthy human interaction and connection, and the vast majority of recovering sex addicts can't simply abstain or even significantly limit their use of it. The good news is that sex addicts can now fight fire with fire, installing "parental-control software" on their digital devices.

As the parental-control label suggests, these products were initially developed to protect children from unwanted online content and contacts. However, as the products have become more sophisticated over time, they have also become more versatile, and many are now quite useful to adults who struggle with online behaviors, including sexual behaviors.

Generally speaking, parental-control software products offer a combination of filtering/blocking and monitoring/accountability. The filtering portions of these programs offer variations of the following:

- Customizable website filtering and blocking
- Online search filtering and blocking
- App filtering and blocking
- Social media blocking
- Instant message/chat blocking
- File transfer blocking (preventing the sending and receiving of pictures, videos, and the like)
- Video game filtering
- Profanity blocking

The accountability features of these products typically include variations of the following:

- Regular and on-demand reports (for the accountability partner)
- Real-time alerts if the sex addict uses or attempts to use a digital device in a prohibited way
- Log of websites visited
- Log of online searches
- Log of social networking sites utilized
- Log of usernames and passwords
- Log or transcript of IM and chat activity
- Log or transcript of email activity
- Screenshot playbacks

It is important to state that filtering and accountability products are not guarantees of sexual sobriety. In truth, a persistent or tech-savvy sex addict can nearly always find ways to circumvent even the best of these products. And if the software stumps an addict, he or she can just go out and buy a new digital device and then use it in secret. As such, filtering and accountability products should not be viewed as enforcers of recovery; instead, they should be looked at as a tool of recovery that can help sex addicts maintain sobriety by reducing impulsive online behavior (through the filtering and blocking features) and rebuild trust (through the accountability and reporting features). Unsurprisingly, some of these products are better than others; annually updated reviews are posted on the website of the Sexual Recovery Institute at: sexualrecovery.com/online-controls-for-sex-romance-addicts/.

AFTERWORD

Sexual fantasies and activities are one of several paths to enjoyment, play, and personal relationship for the majority of us. Sexual addicts, on the other hand, engage in these behaviors compulsively, eventually losing control and having to deal with negative life consequences as a result. Because of their addiction, their belief systems, self-esteem, and relationships suffer. Happily, the definition of sexual sobriety does not include total abstinence. Instead, sex addicts must, like people who struggle with eating disorders, find a way to healthfully integrate this naturally important element of life into their day-to-day existence. This book provides sexual addicts (and those who care about them) with a road map for doing this.

Over the last several decades, countless thousands of sex addicts and their loved ones have found recovery and healing by following the steps outlined herein: under-standing and recognizing their problem, visiting a knowl-edgeable sex-addiction treatment specialist, getting involved in twelve-step and related support groups, dealing with concurrent disorders related to their addiction, setting appropriate boundaries for sex, dating, and relationship integrity, rebuilding their relationships, and restoring balance and freedom to their lives. The best part is that getting started is extremely easy. All that is needed is a willingness to be transparent and honest about one's situation and to seek support.

Suppose you are sexually addicted, or you think that someone you know and care about is sexually addicted. In that case, I hope you have found this book both enlightening and helpful and that you feel motivated to undertake the process of recovery, healing, and a more meaningful, connected, and rewarding life. If so, everything you need to get well is out there waiting for you to get started. I wish you the very best of luck on your journey.

REFERENCES

A. Cooper, D. E. Putman, L. A. Planchon, and S. C. Boies, "Online
    Sexual Compulsivity: Getting Tangled in the Net,"
Sexual Addiction and Compulsivity 6 (1999): 79–104.

Adams, K. M. (2011). Silently Seduced: When parents make their
    children partners. Health Communications, Inc.

American Psychiatric Association (2013). Diagnostic and statistical
    manual of mental disorders: DSM-5. Washington, D.C.:
American Psychiatric Association.

American Psychological Association. "Sexual orientation and
    homosexuality," apa.org/helpcenter/,accessed March 30,
2021.

Carnes, P. (1989). Contrary to love: Helping the sexual addict. Center
City, MN: Hazelden.

Carnes, P. (1991). Don't call it love: Recovery from sexual addiction.
New York, NY: Bantam.

Carnes, P. (2001). Out of the shadows: Understanding sexual addiction
(3rd Ed.). Center City, MN:Hazelden.

Carnes, P. (1983). Out of the Shadows: Understanding Sexual
Addiction (1st Edition). Center City, MN:Hazelden.

Cooper, A. (1998). Sexuality and the Internet: Surfing into the new
millennium. CyberPsychology & Behavior, 1(2), 187–193.

"Definition of Addiction," American Society of Addiction Medicine,
accessed March 27, 2021, asam.org/for-the-public/definition-of-addiction.

Goldman, D., Oroszi, G., & Ducci, F. (2005). The genetics of
addictions: uncovering the genes. Nature Reviews Genetics, 6(7), 521–532.

Hall, P. (2013). Understanding and treating sex addiction: A comprehensive guide for people who struggle with sex addiction and those who want to help them, p 15. London: Routledge.

Hall, P. (2013). Understanding and treating sex addiction: A
comprehensive guide for people who struggle with sex addiction and those who want to help them, pp 51–60. London: Routledge.

Hall, P. (2013). Understanding and treating sex addiction: A
comprehensive guide for people who struggle with sex addiction and those who want to help them, p 40. London: Routledge.

Matt, F. (2017). The Porn Myth: Exposing the Reality Behind the
Fantasy of Pornography. Ignatius Press

Robert, W. (2015). Sex Addiction 101: A Basic Guide to Healing from
Sex, Porm, and Love Addiction. Health Communications, Inc.

Wilson, G. (2014). Your Brain on Porn: Internet Pornography and the
Emerging Science of Addiction. Richmond, VA: Commonwealth Publishing.

Wolak, J., Mitchell, K., & Finkelhor, D. (2007). Unwanted and wanted exposure to online pornography in a national sample of youth Internet users. Pediatrics, 119(2), 247–257.

Made in the USA
Las Vegas, NV
15 June 2024

91099110R00129